Healthcare as a Universal Human Right

This important book outlines how, despite varying levels of global socioeconomic development, governments around the world can guarantee their citizens' fundamental right to basic healthcare.

Grounded in the philosophical position that healthcare is an essential element to human dignity, the book moves beyond this theoretical principle to offer policy-makers a basis for health policies based on public accountability and social responsiveness. Also emphasizing the importance of global cooperation, particularly in the area of health promotion and communication, it addresses, too, the issue of financial sustainability, suggesting robust mechanisms of economic and social regulation. New opportunities created by e-health, evidence-based data, and artificial intelligence are all highlighted and discussed, as is the issue of patient rights.

Students and researchers across bioethics, public health, and medical sociology will find this book fascinating reading, as will policy-makers in the field.

Rui Nunes is a full professor of bioethics at the Faculty of Medicine of the University of Porto. He is the president and founder of the Portuguese Association of Bioethics and is a member of the Portuguese National Council of Ethics for Life Sciences. He has published nearly 30 books in different areas. He got international recognition due to the proposal in Brazil and Portugal of the legalization of the living will and due to the proposal to UNESCO of the Universal Declaration on Gender Equality. Between 2016 and 2021 he was the Head of the Research Department of the International Network of the UNESCO Chair in Bioethics. He is the Secretary-General of the International Chair in Bioethics.

Healthcare as a Universal Human Right

Sustainability in Global Health

Rui Nunes

Routledge
Taylor & Francis Group

LONDON AND NEW YORK

First published 2022
by Routledge
4 Park Square, Milton Park, Abingdon, Oxon OX14 4RN

and by Routledge
605 Third Avenue, New York, NY 10158

Routledge is an imprint of the Taylor & Francis Group, an informa business

© 2022 Rui Nunes

The right of Rui Nunes to be identified as author of this work has been asserted in accordance with sections 77 and 78 of the Copyright, Designs and Patents Act 1988.

British Library Cataloguing-in-Publication Data
A catalogue record for this book is available from the British Library

Library of Congress Cataloging-in-Publication Data
A catalog record for this book has been requested

ISBN: 978-1-032-13880-0 (hbk)
ISBN: 978-1-032-19325-0 (pbk)
ISBN: 978-1-003-24106-5 (ebk)

DOI: 10.4324/9781003241065

Typeset in Goudy
by Apex CoVantage, LLC

Contents

Figures

Boxes

Acknowledgments

The author thanks Guilhermina Rego, Cristina Brandão, and Sofia B. Nunes for their valuable contributions and insights to this book and for the coauthorship of some of the papers that were instrumental for its edition. This book was published under the patronage of the PhD Program in Bioethics of the Faculty of Medicine of the University of Porto.

Introduction

In many societies, the right to access healthcare is considered a positive welfare right and it may very well be one of the most important achievements of modern democracies; that is, it is a right drawn from civilization itself and an expression of the dignity of a human being. Then, one may deduce that the right to access healthcare is decisive for exercising a fair equality of opportunity in a free and inclusive society. Indeed, disease, disability, and incapacity restrict opportunities that would otherwise be available to the individual. These situations must be observed as unjust and not just as the result of random forces of nature.

However, if it is true that many developed societies fulfill this right, there is variability in this area (namely in the structure of the healthcare system), and since this right is inherent to the human condition, one may ask whether it should be enjoyed by all people in all countries of the world. This book presents a theoretical construct that allows the implementation of the right to healthcare of appropriate quality on a global scale, regardless of the specific economic and social circumstances within each society. Indeed, universal health coverage can be implemented worldwide if the specific level of coverage is indexed to the level of resources (human, material, and technological) available in any specific society.

To materialize the proposal of a universal right to healthcare, and therefore, to universal health coverage, here, an attempt was made to reconcile John Rawls' social contract theory and Norman Daniels' accountability for reasonableness with the global justice vision of Amartya Sen. The universal right to healthcare means universal health coverage for all people, regardless of the country of residence. This book does not intend to suggest the creation of supranational structures to enforce this right to healthcare. Rather, the realization of this right must take place pragmatically in each nation-state using its endowed resources, notwithstanding eventual support from the international community. In a realistic way, this proposal is in accordance with the sovereignty of every nation-state, namely regarding its social and economic choices and the level of development of the welfare state.

Despite a gradual improvement in humanity's living conditions, large disparities still exist between and within countries regarding human development indicators because of economic globalization and a climate of international prosperity. If we consider that Sen's human development index (a proxy for the human condition

DOI: 10.4324/9781003241065-1

and development) combines per capita income indicators with life expectancy and education, then universal access to the healthcare system and its translation into health outcomes is also a decisive factor for full human development (for instance, as in the inequality-adjusted human development index). First, this index is a central element in the fight against poverty and different social inequalities. Hence, sustainable human development goes beyond wealth creation and implies, for instance, enhancing equity, empowerment of different social groups, and appropriately managing the demographic transition besides promoting environmental protection.

This book intends to present a pragmatic view of international relations and domestic public policies assuming that despite the existence of global governance institutions in politics (e.g., United Nations (UN)), education (e.g., United Nations Educational, Scientific, and Cultural Organization (UNESCO)), health/healthcare (e.g., World Health Organization (WHO)), economic and financial systems (e.g., the World Bank System (WB) and the International Monetary Fund (IMF)), and even with regard to free international trade (e.g., World Trade Organization (WTO)), there are no comprehensive mechanisms for global implementation of human rights. It is not expected to exist such comprehensive mechanisms in the near future. Thus, in the absence of effective global governance and sufficiently robust international institutions, it is important to find adequate solutions to achieve one of the greatest human aspirations: the satisfaction of basic health needs. Most advanced democracies have already accomplished this goal, and these examples may be reproduced and even enhanced in most countries.

Notably, the international community has committed itself to the implementation of transnational policies in healthcare. For example, there are important efforts to promote global health, namely preventing infectious diseases or other global threats, such as COVID-19. The global economic impact of many diseases, besides the huge distress caused by the mobility of people worldwide, justifies transnational public health measures. Indeed, transnational healthcare cooperation is perfectly compatible with the national implementation of a modern healthcare system and the promotion of global health measures to promote health worldwide. This is because no nation is capable by itself in accomplishing global health endeavors.

An integrated view of the main theories of distributive justice based on the substantive ethical principles of personal freedom, fair equality of opportunity, and solidarity is presented with the aim of demonstrating that every human being should enjoy the best possible conditions for normal performance in society. All societies face resource scarcity and, therefore, must take adequate measures to ensure access to healthcare. I suggest that any proposal for the implementation of universal health coverage must be based on an "ethical platform," namely on the principles of fair equality of opportunity in access, solidarity in financing, effectiveness of interventions, and efficiency in resource allocation (value for money).

The instruments (economic and financial) guaranteeing the pursuit of fair equality of opportunity are not particularly relevant to the discussions in this book. It is even irrelevant whether the financing of the health system is essentially based on taxes, as is the case in the United Kingdom (Beveridge type systems) or compulsory public insurance according to the citizens' income, as is the case in Germany (Bismarck type systems). Rather, on the one hand, what is at issue is universal access to healthcare of appropriate quality, and on the other hand, the equitable distribution of resources at a territorial level. An egalitarian dimension of justice in the context of resource allocation for health may imply an acceptable (or reasonable) level of healthcare provision. Depending on whether a basic package is implemented, healthcare levels should allow for the delivery of appropriate preventive and curative medicine. However, in principle, different levels of provision and access depending on individual income are admissible (tiering), but only when access to the basic level is guaranteed for all citizens.

There are several alternative models for implementing universal health coverage. However, in all systems, the establishment of priorities in healthcare is progressively implemented. This is because in public systems, it is not possible to control the demand for healthcare. Therefore, rationing must be implemented, either implicitly or explicitly, in accordance with ethical and legal standards. For the establishment of priorities in healthcare to be considered fair and equitable, public preferences must be legitimized. The sources of legitimacy (substantive and not merely formal) can come from two different ways: a) the popular preferences expressed through the democratic vote in specific elections and b) direct involvement and participation of society. This empowerment of society for collective purposes implies a wide base of support so that the absence of citizens' votes can be filled by an adequate, comprehensive, and transparent deliberation.

Ultimately, it is a matter of procedural justice that includes fair, responsive, and transparent procedures under society's supervision. Therefore, public accountability is an ethical imperative in any advanced democracy. While procedural justice – as the common denominator of most distributive justice theories – may not be the best, it is the only solution in a society in which citizens are moral strangers and in which there is no unanimous view of the common good. Therefore, the rationale for the establishment of priorities should have broad participation of all stakeholders involved in these decisions. Thus, to be legitimate, appropriate solutions must be found to achieve the legitimacy of this type of decision. That is, both accountability and responsiveness are important principles of modern public policy.

Prioritizing healthcare implies that in any society, a previous effort to rationalize resources (so that inefficiency is minimal) is made; therefore, it is fair and appropriate to make choices that are accountable and responsive. Indeed, there is an equation that combines public services with public sector and public spending in accordance with a view of public service ethos. However, public choice theorists have challenged traditional modalities of public administration because frequent public interest is not accomplished, as seen by the growing inefficiency and government failures in many sectors, such as healthcare and education. The new public management in healthcare is in accordance with this perspective to promote efficiency and equity in access to the health system. However, new public management is not the only new way to manage public services.

New public management implies that new management modalities are implemented and that competition is the basis of the system. "Government by contract," in which public hospitals compete between themselves by public financing, is the paradigm of this entrepreneurial culture. This government by contract is closely connected to the implementation of an internal, administrative market (quasi market) in the public system within which public providers (although of a corporate nature) also compete with private providers for public financing. The corporatization of public hospitals is the rule through the introduction of private tools of management in the public sphere. In addition, strategic planning of health services is implemented to achieve a long-term balance in the provision of healthcare facilities. The private finance initiative, in which private corporations run public hospitals, is another good example of this evolution.

This evolution is also accomplished through the emergence of a "regulatory state," as suggested by Giandomenico Majone. Indeed, the regulatory state is an example of this systematic change in public administration in which the government guarantees citizens' rights, but in which different providers from the public and private sectors coexist. The rise of independent regulation is also a distinctive feature of the regulatory state, namely through the creation of Independent Regulatory Agencies (IRAs). The objective of these agencies is to promote economic and social regulation and prevent discriminatory practices against patients, namely cream skimming of expensive diseases that are not profitable and stimulating a fair and competitive internal market in healthcare. In this way, the system will be more efficient and healthcare quality will also be promoted, thereby guaranteeing equity in access to a competitive and universal public system.

Modern healthcare systems improve efficiency in resource allocation and provide value for money through the promotion of primary healthcare and preventive measures. Indeed, primary care fulfills the dual function of gatekeeping (rationalization of the demand for hospital care by limiting it to specific cases) and signposting (ability to orient and guide the patient through the health system). Thus, based on the assumption that primary care represents the patient's first contact with the health system, it is important to highlight the crucial role that this level of care plays in promoting health.

It is not just a question of curative care; rather, according to the Declaration of Alma-Ata, it is an approach to the main health problems of a community via health promotion and prevention (primary, secondary, tertiary, and quaternary), and patient treatment and rehabilitation. This declaration emerged from a conference held in Alma-Ata (Kazakhstan) sponsored by the WHO and the United Nations Children's Education Fund (UNICEF), which aimed at highlighting the importance of primary healthcare besides emphasizing its vital importance in any healthcare system. Primary care presupposes a global vision of health along with curative medicine and rehabilitation. Primary care is fulfilled through a well-defined strategy: a) educate for health promotion and disease prevention; b) promote education for responsible sexuality; c) provide maternal and child care and family planning programs; d) promote healthy eating and nutrition; e) guarantee basic sanitary conditions; f) implement mandatory vaccination programs; g) prevent endemic diseases in the population; and h) ensure access to necessary medicines.

Consequently, what is at stake is a horizontal integration of the healthcare system to implement a true preventive medicine attitude with respect to the social and environmental determinants of health. Thus, primary care should be developed at the level of health maintenance, prevention of disease, disease diagnosis and treatment, and patient rehabilitation. Intersectoral efforts are necessary to fulfill these objectives because health gains depend not only on the healthcare system but also on other fundamental areas, such as education, social security, and environmental protection.

Due to the astonishing rise of digital health as a direct consequence of new and modern information and communications technology (ICT), it will be easier to promote integration of the health system and full delivery of healthcare services on a global scale. Although ICT evokes special ethical questions (namely, the duty to protect personal privacy as a basic and irreducible right), it will be instrumental in a modern healthcare system because of the possibility of delivering quality healthcare services even in remote geographical areas via e-health. The interoperability of different systems is a fundamental tool for promoting interconnectivity, which is the cornerstone of this evolution.

However, the existence of large collections of data, both structured and unstructured, also termed big data or even lake data, questions society and public authorities about the destiny of this large amount of information and how it can be used to make better decisions for mankind. Data mining, machine learning (including deep and reinforcement learning), machine reasoning, and robotics (integration of different techniques into cyber-physical systems) have been developed to extract information and transform these data into valuable use in the healthcare system. Artificial intelligence also has a profound impact in modern systems because of the capacity to integrate all this big data and propel it to promote new treatment modalities, besides preventing life-threatening diseases. Indeed, it may help physicians in the diagnosis and treatment of many diseases, and in the real-time monitoring of patients, sometimes at long distances.

Patients, as citizens, have rights and duties in modern societies. Democratic and basic rights of citizenship are frequently ascribed to people in different societies. Healthcare access is one such right. Other rights, such as the right to self-determination or the right to privacy, have gradually become valued worldwide. In addition, the principle of nondiscrimination is paramount so that no one should be discriminated against because of a particular condition, namely gender, age, ethnicity, cultural identity, political affiliation, and other factors. Indeed, human rights are indivisible by nature, meaning that all rights ascribed to an individual should be completely fulfilled, in any circumstance, and especially when they are most vulnerable.

The consideration of special protections for the chronically and terminally ill is unsurprising due to the overall sociodemographic transition of most societies along with the growing impact of chronic diseases. Their inclusion in the healthcare system is progressive and unquestionable. Indeed, palliative care intends to provide global care and spiritual support to the patient and their family when medicine cannot cure the patient's disease. Palliative care, although different in nature compared to acute care, should therefore be considered a huge priority in healthcare. Modern systems should embrace the possibility of creating national and even supranational networks so that elderly and chronic patients find a humane and peaceful way to live and that resources are conveyed to those most in need. Then, universal access to palliative care is a logical evolution of the proposal of healthcare access as a universal right. Consequently, healthcare professionals' education should also be revisited to include a comprehensive curriculum on education for chronic and palliative care even after graduation from their respective programs in conjunction with education for ethics and human rights. This can help medicine and healthcare become even more compassionate despite all their astonishing technological advances.

In short, globalization demands international cooperation to solve health problems that cannot be addressed by individual countries (global health). The COVID-19 pandemic is a good example. However, the fingerprint of a new world political philosophy is to empower countries to implement citizens' basic rights. In the absence of a global civil society and a common shared ideal of world citizenship, we can opt for a pragmatic strategy without renouncing the essence of fundamental rights. The supranational European project is an important effort to create a planetary consciousness about the primacy of the person and of the ideal of a "minimal humanitarianism." In the future, this ideal of freedom can lead to a global humanitarian identity.

Indeed, the pillar of modern and developed societies is that all people have equal dignity and should be able to enjoy a broad set of basic, inalienable, and indivisible rights. This fundamental equality among all human beings was the basis of the construction of the charter of human rights and is the most important unifying agent of humanity on a global scale. Perhaps that charter is why the right to health is now considered a right of civilization. This right clearly implies universal health coverage that encompasses at least an adequate minimum care. However, prioritizing healthcare delivery and promoting efficiency by properly managing financial, human, and material resources are also needed. Moreover, resources for providing adequate care to the population, besides subsequent rationing, should also be carried out under the criteria of accountability, responsibility, and responsivity.

It is in this conceptual framework that the implementation of a universal right to healthcare access on a global scale is proposed, while always keeping in mind that a healthy society is more cohesive and productive. This perspective may contribute to a more prosperous, peaceful, and sustainable world.

1 Fair Equality of Opportunity in Healthcare[1]

The allocation of resources for health, besides the distribution of other social goods, is a political problem. It can also be observed as belonging to the universe of distributive justice, in which all citizens must have the necessary means for an acceptable physical, psychological, and social performance. Individual autonomy, which is the paradigm of full citizenship in a modern society, cannot otherwise be achieved. However, the principle of solidarity, as an ethical and social imperative, can also be invoked to protect the worse-off members of society. The principle of solidarity via the tax effort of citizens can allow a balanced allocation of resources in society. In Europe, the Convention on Human Rights and Biomedicine (Council of Europe 1996) promotes this ideal by appealing to a universal right of access to healthcare. The ethical and social implications of this convention may determine the acceptance of this right as a fundamental one in accordance with the Universal Declaration of Human Rights.

Indeed, in most civilized countries, the welfare state formula promoted by Bismarck transformed the ideal of justice into an integral element of social and community life. The acceptance of health as a social good brought about a health protection policy that was adapted to this perspective (Ruger 2004). However, the welfare state crisis, mainly related to the increase in life expectancy and the increase in the costs of providing healthcare (mainly due to scientific and technological progress), suggested a different approach to this problem. It generated the urgent need to establish priorities in healthcare (Wilson 2018). Moreover, the overall improvement of the population's living conditions (at a social, cultural, educational, and economic level) is responsible for the sustained evolution of health indicators in developed countries together with the provision of medical care.

Nowadays, and in a global society, citizens are more critical of their healthcare systems due to the information obtained through different channels of communication. Information regarding new treatment methods and sophisticated technology is rapidly being introduced into the health market. Thus, we must review the very concept of *right of access to healthcare*: if the demand for healthcare based on individual needs is unlimited, it is essential to limit the supply and, therefore, access to healthcare. However, the methods that lead to the establishment of

DOI: 10.4324/9781003241065-2

priorities must be transparent and previously legitimized by the democratic process (Nunes and Rego 2014).

Equal Opportunity: An Aspirational Value?

A priori, one may question the plausible justification for fundamental equality between all persons (Sen 1999). This equality could be because all people belong to the human moral community, owing the obligation of support and solidarity to each other. In essence, the human being is a relational being who is living and interacting constantly with their fellow citizens. This is not to say that all people are equal in the strictest sense of the term. In fact, we are all biologically and intellectually different. Indeed, rationality is the supreme attribute of the human species and distinguishes and characterizes everyone's personality. Moreover, true social equality at all levels and in all contexts is perhaps an intangible reality. The concept of equality refers to the inclusion in a group that gives equal rights to all its members, at least regarding certain basic and fundamental rights.

This concept does not imply behavior standardization; uniformity is opposed to the very essence of human nature, given that intellectual creativity is a factor that argues in favor of the existence of the moral community itself. Thus, there will always be differences between people, regardless of their fundamental rights. The inalienable rights to life, food, constitution of family, and access to healthcare do not imply that everyone is the same nor that they have the same ambitions to carry out the same life projects. It implies that whatever their intellectual skills may be and hence, their ability to flourish within society, they are guaranteed a reasonable level of social conditions consistent with the dignity of the human being. This principle of equal dignity of human beings seems to be decisive in the implementation of a policy of fair equality of opportunity with respect to access to social goods.

However, note that different aspects of justice have a general application regarding the distribution of wealth and property. Society, regardless of the diversity of cultures and traditions within it, is generally organized around a state with rules of social coexistence, which are translated into the creation and approval of own orders in the ethical and legal sphere. According to Thomas Hobbes, the organization of the state is based on the assumption that human beings are constantly fighting for survival, as they are according to the law of nature, "the enemy of every human being" (Hobbes [1651] 1994). In fact, the constant search for happiness requires a human being to always desire more power and, therefore, more wealth as a guarantee of their survival. Thus, power implies more power, always at the expense of other human beings. Happiness is observed as the continuous progression of individual desire and is also achievement beyond possessions. This innate desire among human beings to always wish for more power leads the human community to organize itself via civil laws to ensure its survival.

Hobbes further argues that this natural situation of the social man is only possible because in the natural state, human beings are very similar to each other within physical and spiritual spheres. This natural equality among human beings has three aspects: a) agency/competence; b) mutual mistrust; and c) the desire for success. It is also argued that these decisions have nothing to do with just or unjust, given that the concept of justice does not fit into the biological evolution of humanity. The institutional creation of the state by mutual agreement seeks to prevent the process of self-destruction of humans by humans. The state, *civitas* in Latin, derives from this human social pact that was created by and for humans by exercising its power according to the sovereign will of those it represents. However, an idea of the state as a centralized and maximalist structure of power can be clearly contradicted, not in the sense of anarchic coexistence but in the sense of a minimalist state or a limited government. This government seeks to guarantee sovereignty and public order but allows individual energies to have free expression, thus ensuring social cohesion. Hence, the importance of a social protection system, including access to healthcare, can be upheld.

Norman Daniels refers to the social obligation through the government's direct intervention to provide healthcare, based on the "normal functioning" standard (Daniels 1985). Universality of healthcare access should be promoted to guarantee each citizen's access to a normal performance and, therefore, to a reasonable range of social opportunities. In this perspective of justice, the existence of disease, disability, and incapacity are observed as unfair and not just as the result of random forces of nature as they restrict the opportunities that would otherwise be available to the individual. From this viewpoint, one may deduce that the right of access to healthcare is decisive for exercising fair equality of opportunity. That is, the right to healthcare access imposes a duty on society to allocate resources according to its citizens' health needs (World Health Organization 1996).

The conviction that fair and equal opportunity for citizens reflects the need to ensure "normal," but not necessarily "equal," performance should be emphasized. This distinction is fundamental since no person is equal to another in a strict sense. In fact, all citizens should have the right of access in accordance with their intrinsic dignity to certain essential goods so that it is possible to at least guarantee a reasonable physical, psychological, and social performance. Thus, talents and individual capacities are likely to be achieved, even if only in specific circumstances.

However, equal opportunity may be limited by resource scarcity in society if the choices in healthcare delivery are transparent, public, and periodically submitted to an audit process in accordance with democratic rules (Daniels et al. 1996). This perspective of distributive justice is based on the notion of democratic accountability. It justifies the scope and limitations of the provision of healthcare services. According to Daniels (1998), the concept of procedural justice may imply transparency and accountability in the context of provisioning healthcare (Daniels 1998). Citizens have the right to be informed about the reasons that led to the establishment of priorities. This concept of public accountability assumes that decisions are not only transparent and democratic but also taken in accordance with what "reasonable people" would decide under different sets of circumstances (Nunes and Rego 2014).

According to Wikler and Marchand (1998), society's intervention is growing with respect to the macro-allocation of resources for provisioning healthcare. This is partly due to the lack of consensus on the principles by which this allocation should be guided. Again, democratic accountability and its practical application seem to be the most transparent way of applying the principle of justice, at least as far as procedural justice is concerned, although theoretically, it may not be the ideal of distributive justice. In this context, access to new technologies, such as innovative and expensive treatments, can be legitimately restricted but only if this decision is determined by society and imposed by financial constraints of the system.

To achieve fair equality of opportunity, it is fundamental to promote the values in which a society that is constantly changing can contribute to this ideal of distributive justice. In the field of healthcare access, solidarity in financing and equity in access have been proposed. Equity can refer also to *equality of liberty*, indicating that in a more economic than philosophical sense, it can be said that everyone prefers to decide on the allocation of resources instead of accepting what was proposed by another person. Of course, an assumption will be that the individual has the necessary means to make that choice. Thus, equity includes the concept of equality in individual self-actualization (Parijs 1991).

Achieving equity in access to social goods implies a systematic reduction of disparities between individual citizens and different social groups. One of the main factors leading to the overall improvement in population health lies both in the reduction of cultural, economic, and social disparities between the best and the worst-off citizens and in the quality of health services. As a political and ideological option, the concept of equity can have different social and economic implications: a) equity in the resource allocation; b) equity in the provision of healthcare; and c) equity in the payment of healthcare.

The application of the principle of justice can give rise to a distinction between horizontal and vertical equities. Horizontal equity means the provision of equal treatment to equal individuals. Vertical equity presupposes unequal treatment for unequal individuals. Therefore, it is possible to determine relevant properties in individuals who give expression to this perspective of justice (Beauchamp and Childress 2013) and thus, promote vertical equity. In this context, justice is perhaps related to the concepts of *necessity* and *normal functioning*, which are possibly the starting points for an equal opportunity policy. The adoption of measures conducive to vertical equity intends to meet the well-documented sociological reality that the worse-off citizens, based on the economic point of view, are also those with the worst health indicators (Chisholm 2018).

However, in market economies, solidarity does not materialize on purely altruistic grounds to achieve equity in the access and distribution of social goods. If *solidarity* means the perception of unity and the will to suffer the consequences thereof, the concept of *unity* indicates the presence of a group of people with a common history and with similar values and convictions. According to the Report by the Government Committee on Choices in Health Care (1992), "Solidarity can be voluntary, as when people behave out of humanistic motives, or compulsory as when the government taxes the population to provide services to all." Again, in most modern democracies, the state feels the need to find ways to guarantee the fundamental rights of citizens through the tax structure. Indeed, when human beings are free from ignorance and fear and when the standard of living increases steadily, they evolve similarly to freedom and interpersonal solidarity.

Solidarity has different backgrounds from a historical viewpoint. Although with different names, solidarity can be found in different religious traditions and in Marxism, socialist, and even liberal thought. As a doctrine or as a political choice, solidarity is deeply rooted in most healthcare systems. The pursued social good (health), not only for the individual but also for society, in addition to the symbolic value that disease has for everyone, implies state intervention to ensure access to a certain level of healthcare. Solidarity in health can also contribute to another social function. Solidarity can generate solidarity due to the *moral movement of society* (Brandão et al. 2013). A good example is the creation of a universal public health system as a source of altruism that usually extends to other areas of society.

It is also necessary to distinguish between intra- and intergenerational solidarity. As an example, promoting the welfare of young generations is the best way to guarantee a stable support network (namely through a healthy productive force) for future generations. Thus, guaranteeing the right to an open future for the young generations is a win-win strategy. That is why it is difficult to accept any strategy that is intergenerationally disruptive, such as the "fair innings" theory. This theory states that justice in resource allocation should be related to the number of years lived with the fair share of the social resources already consumed along with the provision of medical care (Williams 1994). According to this perspective, as life expectancy in modern countries is over 80 years, society's responsibility to provide healthcare would be inversely proportional to the number of years lived. Beyond the average life expectancy, society would no longer have the responsibility of providing healthcare to elderly citizens.

A strictly utilitarian view contributes to this theoretical arrangement because by giving preference to programs of preventive health to the young generations, we are increasing the number of *years-benefit* and therefore, the overall well-being of society. For example, Daniel Callahan (1987) argues that society must provide the means for children to reach old age and only use the scarce financial resources so that the elderly can become even older when that goal is achieved. However, in the long run, the social impact of these measures can contribute to the disintegration of society by excluding entire groups of citizens from basic healthcare, which is precisely what utilitarianism seeks to avoid.

However, there are huge global disparities in the quantity of resources that can be allocated to healthcare delivery. Hence, a variable geometry may imply a conceptual reframing and an adjustment of the application of these principles according to the concrete reality of each society (Buchanan 2000). This is notwithstanding the fact that global health implies both strategy and coordination at a global level and the implementation of healthcare systems in every sovereign state in the world (Meier and Gostin 2018; Gostin and Meier 2020).

Progressive Justice

There are different conceptual roots regarding the concept of justice in resource allocation for the provision of healthcare. Various theories invariably appeal to the formal principle of justice that *equals* should be treated *in the same way in the exact measure of its similarity or dissimilarity* (formal equality principle of Aristotle). This principle is called formal because it outlines the arrangements of justice between citizens, although it does not allow us to deduce which substantive differences make citizens equals or not equal.

The lack of substance of this formal principle is revealed by the fact that it is not possible to specify the relevant properties or circumstances of the subject that allow the determination of this equality. It is precisely to incorporate "substance" into the "form" proposed by Aristotle that different theories have proposed different material principles of justice over the centuries (Box 1.1).

Box 1.1   Material Principles of Justice

1   **Radical Egalitarianism**: Identical distribution of social goods by all citizens. For example, access to universal vaccination programs (such as COVID-19).
2   **Necessity**: Access to social goods according to individual needs, meaning equal consideration of the interests of each citizen. For example, access to hospital and prehospital medical emergencies.
3   **Effort**: Access to and distribution of social assets are in line with the effort made by each one. For example, remuneration by medical act in the case of private practice (out of the pocket).
4   **Merit**: Access to scarce goods in society is done according to individual merit. For example, access to the best universities.
5   **Social Contribution**: The contribution of the individual to society is considered decisive (from the economic, family, cultural, or other point of view; for example, the God's Committee, which in Seattle in the 1960s selected patients for kidney dialysis according to socioeconomic status, income level, and the number of descendants).
6   **Competition and Market**: Access to and distribution of social and economic goods in addition to access to key positions in society are made according to the rules of the market. For example, the charges of commercial health insurances.

All social protection systems, particularly access to health, integrate different material principles of justice, sometimes in a contradictory manner, so that the need arose to resort to different "distributive justice theories" to better frame the right of access to healthcare. Through theory, we can understand an integrated and systematized body of rules and principles with internal coherence and logic. The view of distributive justice that confirms most with the conceptual formulation of the welfare state is perhaps the egalitarian theory that rests on the concept of social contract. In the words of John Rawls (1971, 1993), this contract implies that a plural society which is well organized and well structured has individual freedom and fair equality of opportunities in access to social goods as fundamental values.

Rawls defines a theoretical situation in which the impartial observer (reasonable citizen) is on an imaginary plane (ahistoric and acultural) without knowing their financial, cultural, social, health, or illness position (under a veil of ignorance). In this situation, any reasonable citizen would choose to distribute social goods and access to key positions in society so that at the end of the decision-making process, the most disadvantaged people are protected. Thus, Rawls' two principles of justice were formulated, hierarchically, as follows:

1   Every citizen must have access to the most complete system of basic freedoms, including access to key positions in society.
2   This must be carried out on the basis of a fair equality of opportunity basis (and not just on formal equal opportunity).
3   Further, in the end, the allocation of resources and the distribution of social goods should benefit the worse-off in society.

The principle of fair equality of opportunity has become one of the main instruments that determine social policies in the developed world. This justifies some policies of positive discrimination, of which affirmative action in the United States (US) or in Brazil is a good example. In the corresponding policies in these two countries, members of cultural minorities are given priority in access to certain key positions in society (universities for example) or in the implementation of policies on gender equality and protection of the handicapped. The existence of formal institutions legitimated by the public authorities is a direct consequence of this model of social organization as a prerequisite for the widespread implementation of these values. Rawls also refers to the concept of "primary social goods" that every citizen wants himself to achieve self-actualization. First, it is the confirmation of freedom as a fundamental right; second, the fair distribution of socioeconomic benefits; and third, access to these benefits on an equal opportunity basis. In any case, there is a hierarchical order among the principles as freedom is specially valued and protected.

Meanwhile, Ronald Dworkin claims that equality is the main virtue of a sovereign society and true equality means "equality in the value of the resources that each person commands, not in the success he or she achieves" so that modern societies should evolve accordingly (Dworkin 2000). Further, Michael Sandel states that equality means gathering the means to and providing for the social and economic environment for self-realization (Sandel 2009). The specific way in which each person chooses to self-actualize is within the scope of self-determination and is no longer a matter of justice. It is a matter of justice, however, to overcome the unfair circumstances of life determined by the social (familial and social environments) and biological (genetic defects at birth or acquired developmental diseases) lotteries, or to overcome unjust interventions of third parties that seriously limit one's expectations.

However, we can envisage justice arrangements not only as a process (equal opportunity) but as a goal, for instance, human development. Amartya Sen says,

> Development can be seen, it is argued here, as a process of expanding the real freedoms that people enjoy. Focusing on human freedoms contrasts with narrower views of development, such as identifying development with the growth of the gross national product, or with the rise in personal incomes, or with industrialization, or with technological advance or with social modernization. The growth of GNP or individual incomes can, of course, be very important as a *means* of expanding the freedoms enjoyed by the members of the society. But freedoms depend also on other determinants, such as social and economic arrangements (for example, facilities for education and health care) as well as political and civil rights (for example, the liberty to participate in public discussion and scrutiny).
>
> Sen 1999.

Following Sen's account of justice, a global perspective of fairness would

1   promote human freedoms (Sen 1999), and
2   enhance individual capabilities (Sen 1989).

This perspective is a very interesting departure from Rawls' account of justice. Indeed, considering Rawls' first principle of justice (access to most extensive equal liberties for all), this view is morally acquainted with the promotion of a social development system that promotes human freedom. For instance, if I have a) the right and b) the conditions to speak freely, the practical exercise of this right allows me to develop further by effectively using the right. The substantive difference would be that, for Rawls, freedom is a foundational principle of justice (one on which other principles would develop), whereas for Sen, freedom is the overarching goal of social, economic, and political activity (Nunes 2020).

Sen goes even further, stating that

> freedom is central to the process of development for two distinct reasons:
>
> 1 The *evaluative reason*: assessment of progress has to be done primarily in terms of whether the freedoms that people have are enhanced.
> 2 The *effectiveness reason*: achievement of development is thoroughly dependent on the free agency of people.
>
> (Sen 1999)

Thus, full human development requires that basic unfreedoms be effectively outdated (Sen 2009). No one is completely free in the absence of adequate housing, access to basic economic opportunities, access to education and healthcare, or access to basic politic liberties. Interestingly, Rawls' difference principle – protecting the least advantaged social group – combined with the fair equality of opportunity for everyone leads directly (although not in an explicit way) to the enhancement of individual freedoms of the better- and worse-off members of society (Nunes 2020).

For the libertarians such as Robert Nozick (1974), the fundamental values of a democratic society lie in the personal freedom and, for its effective exercise, in the right to private property. It should be noted that libertarianism essentially arises from the field of political philosophy and not from economic theory. Although there is some similarity with the expression "liberalism," they should not be considered equivalent concepts, especially given the economic dimension that is usually associated with the term *liberal*. Freedom of thought, expression, or association overlaps with a utopian vision of equality and social justice. Even so, equal opportunity can be considered an essential tool for the effective exercise of individual freedom. According to this perspective, all people live in a society with a preestablished culture with a history and tradition, in contrast to what was proposed by John Rawls. Moreover, citizens are owners (or not) of property and wealth. These goods are transmitted over the generations. Thus, the coercive expropriation of individual property, namely through taxes, is legitimate but only if it is aimed at obtaining certain social goods (such as public health or national defense) that cannot be left to individual responsibility. The expropriation through taxes is illegitimate if it aims to obtain goods that can be the responsibility of each person, such as health protection or education (not basic).

Whatever social contract exists between the citizens and the state, it must be considered that there are various ways of not complying with tax obligations. Therefore, a contributory/distributive justice is not achieved. On the conceptual plane, the Laffer principle precisely states that beyond a certain level of taxation, taxpayers and institutions find methods for tax evasion which are both legitimate and illegitimate. Thus, pragmatically, greater social justice can be achieved through a lower rate of progressivity in direct taxes. This is based on the idea that most people, by not developing an in-depth system of values, have a distant view of the state only as a guarantor of their rights and not as a source of obligations. Therefore, redistribution of private property through taxes is frequently seen as unfair. The existence of a "distributive justice" is therefore questionable. Moreover, even "contributory justice" (taxes) would be of doubtful legitimacy because the retribution of property according to the criterion of necessity is generally perceived by libertarians as a civilized form of "forced labour" that is only admitted with fiscal consent (Hayek 1976; von Mises 2007).

For example, Tristram Engelhardt Jr. (1996) states that the biological and social lotteries are sometimes considered as a personal and family misfortune; however, their perverse effects are related to neither the notion of justice nor social justice because they do not stem from the intentional action of third parties. Thus, according to libertarians, there is no basic human right of access to healthcare. There could exist a formal right but only if it comes from the freely expressed will of the citizens. For libertarians, healthcare is primarily considered a duty of citizenship, a personal responsibility, and not the government's obligation.

Engelhardt Jr. further argues that postmodern pluralism, which characterizes today's discourse, should consider the divergence of opinion and the fact that any ordering of primary goods is based on certain ethical/philosophical assumptions or a predefined notion of the common good. Therefore, mutual agreement, which is the consent of individuals to common goals, is the only viable instrument for healthy social cooperation between citizens. In this context of intersubjectivity, and even if there is disagreement on the ethical foundation of policy decision-making, it is sufficient to accept common rules of practice to comply with the requirements of procedural justice. Mutual agreement on the procedures to be adopted by citizens can even become a potent cement on a global scale by allowing peaceful coexistence between peoples with distinct cultural traditions. It is only in this way that libertarians will permit the conception of a formal (but not a substantive one) "right" to healthcare.

A third perspective of enormous influence in distributive justice is utilitarianism or existing different backgrounds of this theory that are generally designated by consequentialist or teleological currents. What defines the intrinsic goodness of a social intervention is its purpose and consequences; this is the classic paradigm that the ends justify the means without any proportionality between the two. The main values in question are economic and social efficiency, and the public good. From the methodological viewpoint, the principle of utility can be adopted: an intervention is legitimate if it promotes the greatest possible good for as many people as possible.

Of course, utilitarian strategies favor interventions, such as vaccinations or preventive programs (for instance, vaccination for COVID-19), that target large segments of the population to the detriment of expensive treatments of marginal benefit and limited scope to small groups of citizens. A criticism of utilitarianism is that it allows for discretionary interventions. Discrimination of whole groups of people, such as the disabled, cultural minorities, or the elderly, jeopardizes the principle of intergenerational solidarity and intercultural cohesion. However, from the viewpoint of utilitarianism, a formal right to healthcare access can be shaped, starting from the assumption that utility will be maximized in this way. In fact, a healthy society is a more balanced, stable, and productive one.

Ultimately, this process may involve a genuine procedural justice consisting of fair and transparent procedures under the supervision of society. These procedures, in fact, involve the just acquisition and transfer of property, and the just rectification of the breach of freely celebrated contracts, a reparatory justice of which the criminal justice is a good example. The concept of public accountability should be viewed in this context, wherein there is the need to be accountable for personal and collective decisions (Nunes et al. 2009). Procedural justice, as the common denominator to all the theories of distributive justice, may not be the best. However, it is the only solution in a society in which citizens find themselves with different viewpoints as true "moral strangers" and in which there is no unanimous view of the common good.

The existence of a right to healthcare access should be interpreted in the light of egalitarian theories, namely the principle of fair equality of opportunity and the promotion of personal development and enhanced capabilities. Every citizen must be in the same starting circumstances, biologically and socially, to develop their talents and abilities in accordance with individual autonomy. Further, utilitarian and libertarian values should be considered. On the one hand, the necessary cost control in health and the analyses proposed by health economists of cost-benefit, cost-utility, and cost-effectiveness must be undertaken (Mullen and Spurgeon 2000). On the other hand, the libertarian principles of the autonomy of patients and providers, and freedom of choice and prescription must also be valued in a modern and plural society (Figure 1.1).

However, this interdependent arrangement in resource allocation must consider the hierarchy of individual needs. According to Abraham Maslow's primary and secondary needs (1943), fair equality of opportunities, as an ethical and social

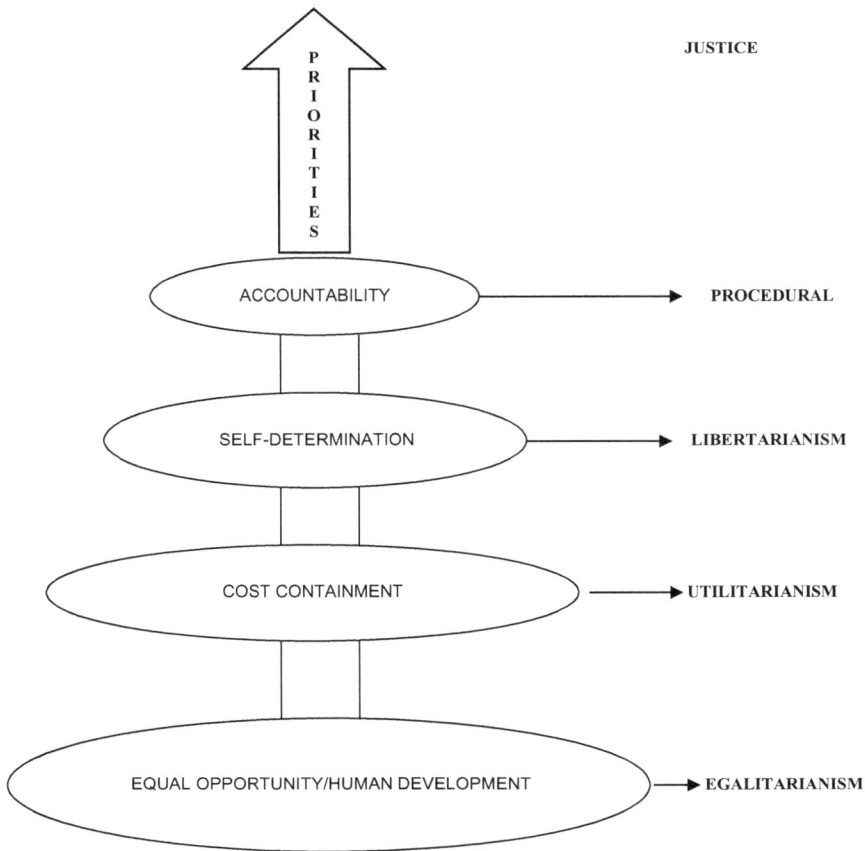

Figure 1.1 Health Protection.

imperative, implies that all citizens must have access to a certain level of conditions that allow them to have *normal functioning*. There are different levels of needs that influence human behavior. Hierarchically superior needs (placed at the top of the pyramid) only manifest themselves when the lower level is satisfied. These lower levels include physiological and safety needs (primary needs). At the higher level, secondary needs (which are social needs) emerge, as does esteem and self-actualization.

Thus, proportionality between the hierarchy of needs in Maslow's pyramid and the concept of normal functioning can be suggested (Nunes and Rego 2014). However, as hierarchically inferior needs are satisfied, the concept of normality becomes more comprehensive, implying its own redefinition. If we consider the fact that "normal" may mean a situation of physical, psychological, and social wellbeing (and perhaps, also spiritual, according to the World Health Organization's definition), it then becomes necessary to satisfy the primary needs to achieve a true equality of opportunities (CIOMS 1997).

Conclusion

Human dignity seems to imply that no citizen can be excluded from the basic healthcare system due to the lack of financial resources. The exercise of individual autonomy, a value specially cherished in plural societies, implies equitable access to certain basic, primary goods, such as healthcare, which are considered essential (Nussbaum 1998). Indeed, equal access of all citizens to basic social goods and, therefore, to key places in society based on the principle of fair equality of opportunities is one of the core aspects of Rawls' difference principle. It is, in essence, about ensuring the exercise of the right to individual self-determination in the relationship between the individual and society, and the right to play a social role according to skills and merit. However, it is not only Rawls' theory of the social contract that describes a fair equality of opportunity. Different perspectives of justice suggest this ideal. Individual autonomy must be interpreted as a value and a determining factor for the exercise of full citizenship. In fact, the poor, the homeless, and the disabled, among others, cannot truly be considered as "equals" regardless of fundamental rights for two reasons: their inability to defend their interests and the vulnerable situation in which they are.

Equity in access to healthcare, as materialized through solidarity in financing and equal opportunity in access, implies that all people with similar health needs should have the same effective opportunity to receive appropriate treatment. However, equity does not imply that in all circumstances there is a social duty to provide for treatment; rather, the specific needs of all citizens are considered in parity and always under the scrutiny of society through the compliance of fair and democratic procedures. Accountability is the guarantor of the exercise of responsibility, at both professional and administrative control levels.

Justice is an ideal that must be progressively built (Nunes et al. 2017). Whether in a specific society or on a global scale, it is a cause and a consequence of full human development. The great challenge of humanity is to precisely recognize the existing intercultural differences and propose sufficiently flexible ideological systems that can be applied in different countries, each with very different levels of social and economic development, without detracting from the ethical principles that should underpin the construction of the 21st-century global society.

Note

1   A previous version of this chapter was published in *Conatus* 3 (2); 2018: 83–97.

References

Beauchamp T and Childress J. 2013. *Principles of biomedical ethics.* Oxford University Press, New York, 7th edition.

Brandão C, Rego G, Duarte I and Nunes R. 2013. Social responsibility: A new paradigm of hospital governance? *Health Care Analysis* 21 (4): 390–402.

Buchanan D. 2000. *An ethic for health promotion. Rethinking the sources of human wellbeing.* Oxford University Press, New York.

Callahan D. 1987. Terminating treatment: Age as a standard. *Hastings Center Report* October–November: 21–25.

Chisholm P. 2018. Preventive healthcare strategies are a matter of social justice. *BMJ* 361: k2699. https://doi.org/10.1136/bmj.k2699.

Choices in Health Care. 1992. *A report by the government committee on choices in health care.* Choices in Health Care, The Netherlands.

CIOMS – Council for International Organizations of Medical Sciences. 1997. *Ethics, equity and health for all*, Z. Bankowski, J. Bryant and J. Gallagher (Editors). CIOMS, Geneva.

Council of Europe. 1996. *Convention for the protection of human rights and dignity of the human being with regard to the application of biology and medicine.* Council of Europe, Strasbourg, November.

Daniels N. 1985. *Just health care. Studies in philosophy and health policy.* Cambridge University Press, New York.

Daniels N. 1998. Is there a right to health care and, if so, what does it encompass? A companion to bioethics. *Blackwell companions to philosophy*, H. Kuhse and P. Singer (Editors). Blackwell Publishers, Oxford.

Daniels N, Light D and Caplan R. 1996. *Benchmarks of fairness for health care reform.* Oxford University Press, New York.

Dworkin R. 2000. *Sovereign virtue. The theory and practice of equality.* Harvard University Press, Cambridge, MA.

Engelhardt HT. 1996. *The foundations of bioethics.* Oxford University Press, New York, 2nd edition.

Gostin L and Meier B (Editors). 2020. *Foundations of global health and human rights.* Oxford University Press, New York.

Hayek FA. 1976. *Law, legislation and liberty. Volume 2. The mirage of social justice.* Routledge & Kegan Paul, London and Henley.

Hobbes T. [1651] (1994). *Leviathan, or the matter, form, and power of a commonwealth, ecclesiastical and civil (1651).* Edwin Curley (Editor), Hackett Publishing, Indianapolis.

Maslow A. 1943. A theory of human motivation. *Psychological Review* July: 370–396.

Meier B and Gostin L. 2018. *Human rights in global health: Rights-based governance for a globalizing world.* Oxford University Press, New York.

Mullen P and Spurgeon P. 2000. *Priority setting and the public.* Radcliffe Medical Press, Abingdon.

Nozick R. 1974. *Anarchy, state and utopia.* Basic Books, New York.

Nunes R. 2020. Addressing gender inequality to promote basic human rights and development: A global perspective. CEDIS Working Papers 2020 (1). http://cedis.fd.unl.pt/blog/project/addressing-gender-inequality-to-promote-basic-human-rights-and-development-a-global-perspective/.

Nunes R, Nunes SB and Rego G. 2017. Healthcare as a universal right. *Journal of Public Health* 25: 1–9.

Nunes R and Rego G. 2014. Priority setting in health care: A complementary approach. *Health Care Analysis* 22: 292–303.

Nunes R, Rego G and Brandão C. 2009. Healthcare regulation as a tool for public accountability. *Medicine, Healthcare and Philosophy* 12: 257–264.

Nussbaum MC. 1998. The good as discipline, the good as freedom. *The ethics of consumption and global stewardship*, D. Crocker D (Editor), 312–341. Rowman and Littlefield, Lanham, MA.

Parijs P. 1991. *Qu'est-ce qu'une société juste? Introduction à la pratique de la philosophie politique.* Éditions du Seuil, Paris.

Rawls J. 1971. *A theory of justice.* Harvard University Press, New York.

Rawls J. 1993. *Political liberalism.* Columbia University Press, New York.

Ruger JP. 2004. Health and social justice. *The Lancet* 364: 1075–1080.

Sandel M. 2009. *Justice: What's the right thing to do?* Farrar, Straus, and Giroux, New York.

Sen A. 1989. Development as capabilities expansion. *The Journal of Development Planning* 19: 41–58.

Sen A. 1999. *Development as freedom.* Knopf, New York.

Sen A. 2009. *The idea of justice.* Harvard University Press, Cambridge.

von Mises L. 2007. *Human action: A treatise on economics.* Liberty Fund Edition, Indianapolis.

Wikler D and Marchand S. 1998. Macro-allocation: Dividing the health care budget. *A companion to bioethics, Blackwell companions to philosophy*, H. Kuhse and P. Singer (Editors). Blackwell Publishers, Oxford.

Williams A. 1994. Economics, society, and health care ethics. *Principles of health care ethics*, R. Gillon (Editor). John Wiley & Sons Ltd, London.

Wilson Y. 2018. Distributive justice and priority setting in health care. *The American Journal of Bioethics* 18 (3): 53–54.

World Health Organization. 1996. *Equity in health and health care.* WHO, Geneva.

2 Welfare State as a Global Ideal

Modern and plural societies base their political regimes on certain basic and inalienable values. These values, namely freedom, equality, and solidarity, are structural elements in the complex relationship between citizens and the state (Rawls 1971). Thus, to realize these rights, several welfare state formulations have been devised over the last century. The core axis of these formulations is the ideal that any person, regardless of their level of income or education level or the result of the biological lottery, should be under the protective sphere of society (Human Development Report 2016). The emergence of social rights, such as the right to access health, education, and/or social protection, is part of this path of solidarity among members of society under equal opportunity conditions (Nagel 1991). The welfare state then emerges as an instrument that aims to guarantee the effective exercise of these rights. The goal is to build a modern, developed, and equitable society. Equal opportunity in access to social goods has been instrumental in achieving this pattern of social interaction (Dworkin 2000).

However, despite a significant improvement in socioeconomic development indicators in modern societies over the last decades, it is necessary to rebuild the welfare state so that it can be a generalizable model on a global scale. On the one hand, *state failures* have been generally demonstrated, whereby some goals of the welfare state are only partially accomplished, even in the most developed countries. On the other hand, the rise in costs associated with social benefits resulting from an aging population increasingly necessitates cost containment. Health and education are paradigmatic examples. The sustainability of public finances implies the reformulation of the welfare state model, which is one of the main problems in modern societies. In fact, the main dilemma of these societies, as denounced by libertarians (Hayek 1976; Nozick 1974), is the difficulty in striking a balance between the duty to provide access to social goods and the establishment of limits imposed by the insurmountable financial constraints on a global scale in which there is a variable geometry of human development.

Therefore, the welfare state, within the context of its various components including health, social security, housing, education, and higher education, should be revisited. This problem is particularly prevalent in weaker economies because of the constraints inherent to their socioeconomic development. In some cases, such as in Europe, the welfare state has progressively developed and has been

DOI: 10.4324/9781003241065-3

reconverted into a smaller and more efficient one. Modern theories in this field converge on the notion that the classical model, which is based on centralized and vertical public administration, is largely outdated. Thus, over the last several years, a dual trend has been observed. On the one hand, some sectors of undeniable socially important economic activity have been privatized, with the understanding that they could be managed more efficiently by the private sector. This privatization is the case with public utilities, such as energy or telecommunications. On the other hand, in sectors in which the state has even greater social responsibilities, the emergence of a new public management and the introduction of competitive internal market mechanisms among providers, including the state as a service provider in the traditional sense of the term, has been observed. This type of system is observable in healthcare.

A fortiori, in this reformist context, one wonders whether the state should be subsidiary in relation to the individual in the protection of goods that may be the latter's responsibility (Nunes et al. 2011). In other words, a new model may have to be considered in which there is an appropriate balance between rights and duties, namely the exercise of responsible citizenship. Political power may then have substantive responsibility to suggest long-term strategies that embody the most fundamental social values of modern societies. Therefore, it is important to evaluate the role of the state in social protection systems to ensure the future viability of these systems.

Modern societies need to reinvent themselves ideologically by finding innovative solutions that allow them to build a sustainable welfare state whose ideological arrangement will have to adjust to the emerging global society and to each society's economy.

A New Social Contract

We now live in a global world. This *global village* is based on the concept of McLuhan and Powers (1989) and brings people together and relativizes distances. The world today is much smaller. Society conveys information in real time by bringing together geographically distant peoples and cultures. However, globalization is not only a result of new information/communication technologies but also the universalization of certain values that are the foundation of contemporary civilization. The acknowledgment of human rights as a fundamental framework and essential level of modern life also implies that values, such as freedom and equal opportunity, are the new language of politics, society, economy, and even international relations (Vasak 1977). This acknowledgment justifies economic freedom, the coexistence of different corporations in a global competitive market, the existence of transnational regulatory mechanisms, or the imposition of certain rules on multinational companies operating in underdeveloped countries that do not respect human rights (such as cases of child labor) (Kumar and Sundarraj 2018).

Then, one may ask how each country can increase the level of wealth, reduce geographical inequities, and adjust the standard of living of the population to fit the country's resources, thus reducing the use of credit with international financial institutions. The successive deficits of many countries and the consequent increase in public debt are the consequence of a confused strategy over the last decades that has not considered the basic principle of budgetary balance. How can we reverse the trend of increasing public debt and the unsustainability of the welfare state with the consequent reduction of resources that can be allocated to the social functions of the state? How can we increase a population's level of human development in a sustainable way?

The implementation of the social market economy is a plausible response to this concept of sustainability, even in the face of economic globalization and huge worldwide competition. The Freiburg School had a profound theoretical and practical influence on the emergence of the social market economy. This school of thought was effervescent in West Germany in the aftermath of World War II. It has had a profound impact on different European countries and is the basis for the creation of the European Union (EU). It is seemingly impossible to reconcile the neoliberal and social-democratic currents that have prevailed in European democracies in the last century. The expression *social market economy* comes from the ordo-economist Alfred Müller-Armack, who reinterpreted the proposals of Walter Eucken, the greatest exponent of the ordo-economy.

> Ordo-liberalism was born in the context of the crisis of the 1920s and 1930s, characterized by huge unemployment, urban violence, great austerity, and an almost ungovernable Weimar Republic. For Walter Eucken, Franz Böhm, Alexander Rüstow, Wilhelm Röpke, and Alfred Müller-Armack, the crisis of that time was the proof that capitalism was unable to subsist economically and politically in an unorganized liberal environment, that is, in an absolute laissez-faire that had brought the more developed countries to unsustainable social conditions.
>
> (Nunes 2013)

Thus, the central idea that presides over the creation of a social market economy is the redefinition of the economic rationality of social relations. Recognizing that collectivist and authoritarian solutions led to the same misery as *unbridled capitalism*, the social market economy assumes that economic freedom underpinning a market economy is the best solution for sustainable economic development and the state should assume the role of disciplining the market.

> For Foucault, ordo-liberalism is an authoritarian liberal project whose purpose is to secure economic freedom by means of a powerful vigilant state action on the economy. The ordo-liberals do not see the market as a self-regulating and self-balanced body as they did not accept the mechanistic view of the neo-classicals. Nor do they see the market as a body. The free economy is created socially, operating with reliance on a permanent and constant political action.
>
> (Nunes 2013)

In addition, ordo-liberalism contrasts partly with libertarianism, which has been defended by authors such as Robert Nozick (1974), and economic liberalism

presented by Ludwig von Mises (2007) and Friedrich Hayek (1976). For libertarians, the fundamental value of a plural society is freedom and for its effective exercise, the right to private property. Freedoms of thought, expression, and
association overlap and, therefore, present a utopian vision of equality and social
justice. From this viewpoint, the compulsory expropriation of individual property
through taxes is legitimate, but only if aimed at obtaining specific social goods,
such as public health (e.g., COVID-19 vaccination) or national defense, which
cannot be left to individual responsibility. In this sense, expropriation through
taxation is illegitimate if the goal is to obtain goods that can be left to individual
responsibility, such as health or education (nonbasic). This laissez-faire, a symbol
of economic liberalism and philosophical libertarianism, was especially valued in
different European countries and the United States in the late nineteenth and
early twentieth centuries and presented itself as an alternative to planned socialist
economies. To some extent, in the genesis of the current economic globalization,
it was the "invisible hand" of the global market.

The social market economy then seeks to situate itself between centralized socialist planning and the unregulated market of laissez-faire liberalism. As
applied by Konrad Adenauer and Ludwig Erhard, this model, which was a merger
of regulated liberalism with the welfare state inherited from Bismarck (Nunes and
Rego 2014), was responsible for the astonishing recovery of the German postwar
economy and created the roots of peace and European unification. The conceptual assumptions of the social market economy propose the implementation of a
macro-socioeconomic model that attempts to reach a consensus of the population around the principles of solidarity and subsidiarity that are necessary for the
survival of this model. Therefore, economic development that requires the accu-
mulation of productive knowledge and its use in both more and more complex
industries would be promoted. In addition, a virtuous combination of functional
capabilities, investment, and innovation through technology would be the driver
of a prosperous economy.

In this model, through some socialization (sometimes only residual) of the
means of production, redistribution of income, equal opportunity in education,
protection of private property, innovation, entrepreneurship, and protection of
social rights, a fair and balanced human development as well as sustainable economic growth would be achieved, always assuming that the government is subsidiary in relation to the more decentralized forms of governance. However, in a
democracy, any model of governance must be legitimized by the social contract
between citizens and the state, and even between the current and the subsequent
generations (Daniels and Sabin 2002). In a developed society, the social contract
must be a pact of association for the construction of a modern and plural society
based on a platform of consensual values among its citizens. This social contract
implies that political and economic freedom always aims to generate a level of
collective well-being that translates into a harmonious growth of society. Social
cohesion must then be a true collective purpose.

Social cohesion implies that within the limits imposed by economic rationality and the available resources, equitable access to certain social benefits and its

multiple components is guaranteed: in education, health, or compensation for loss of income (Power 1997). A concrete application of the principle of equal opportunity is the idea that no citizen should be excluded from the system due to a lack of financial resources. Indeed, one of the pillars of the social market economy is the possibility for all citizens to access social goods under conditions of equal opportunity.

To obtain adequate financing of the welfare state, solidarity is instrumental in redistribution. Solidarity must be understood as

> the awareness of unity and a willingness to bear the consequences of it. Unity indicates the presence of a group of people with a common history and common convictions and ideals. Solidarity can be voluntary, as when people behave out of humanistic motives, or compulsory as when the government taxes the population to provide services to all.
>
> (Choices in Health Care 1992)

Solidarity in financing is generally interpreted through progressivity in taxes and not only through proportionality. While the welfare state's financing is progressive in most societies via direct and indirect taxation, a recurrent criticism of this system is its chronic underfinancing. Samuelson and Nordhaus (2009) establish the following typology of tax revenues:

1   Single rate: for example, a single rate on a particular consumer good, equal for all citizens;
2   Proportional: a fixed value on the income of citizens;
3   Progressive: for example, the variable ranges in the income tax, which increase according to income level; and
4   Regressive: for example, the support given to the financial system by many states, thereby reducing the effective tax rate, to boost productivity, reduce external indebtedness, and thus, stimulate economic growth.

Accepting the principle of tax progressivity as one of the landmarks of a sustainable welfare state and as a means of achieving equity, it is imperative that politically established limits are included. These limits are imposed for two different reasons: a) Arthur Laffer, in 1980, argued that there are direct and indirect mechanisms of tax evasion if the taxpayer perceives the taxes as overrated. Therefore, excessive progressivity will lead to a perverse and counterproductive effect. b) On the basis of John Rawls' (1971) principle of difference, one may argue that the existence of private property (substantially affected if taxes are disproportionate) is an indispensable tool for generating wealth and thus, achieving the goal of protecting the worst-off people. In other words, if the tax system is to be perceived as fair, there must be tax justice not only in combating tax fraud, evasion, and creativity but also in the justice criteria underlying the tax regime.

In any case, global development leads to a demographic transition that is undoubtedly one of the biggest challenges in the welfare state on a global scale.

Improving the population's living conditions has led to an increase in people's longevity and a decrease in the birth rate, with the inevitable inversion of the demographic pyramid. This results in a permanent tension within the welfare state due to the constant need for resources and the impossibility of constantly increasing taxes.

Demographic Transition

Demography is one of the major global challenges of the 21st century. The gradual improvement in socioeconomic living conditions was associated with a considerable decline in the global poverty rate from 37.1% to 9.6% between 1990 and 2015 (The World Bank 2016). This evolution, which is also associated with a universal increase in the quality of healthcare, education, and other social goods, has made it possible for the average life expectancy to grow sustainably throughout the planet over the upcoming decades (Olshansky et al. 2015).

Population aging has also been associated with a reduced birth rate and a significant change in family archetypes. Factors such as family planning, public policies of gender equality (European Commission 2019) with equalization in the labor market, and capabilities expansion (Nunes 2020), or even reduced expectations about the future have led to an inevitable decrease in motivation to procreate. This change dramatically marked the end of the baby boom of the 1950s with a sharp and hardly reversible reduction in the fertility rate in most civilized countries, thus hampering the generational transition itself in most modern democracies. According to the 2018 Aging Report (European Commission 2017), the average life expectancy in 2070 will be 85.9 for men and 90.4 for women; it is estimated that during this century, the average life expectancy may exceed 90 years.

However, these demographic crossroads and the corresponding inversion of the age structure of modern societies have brought new future challenges. For example, the existence of a biotech industrial strategy known as prolongevity (in the framework of the fourth industrial revolution and the digital age) will extend longevity to unimaginable limits (Callahan and Gaylin 2017). Despite the variable geometry in this area, this demographic evolution is expected to be in line with a "longevity dividend" that is fair and consensual via mutual agreement between different generations. This implies that the increase in the average age of the population is directly proportional to improvements in the quality of life at all stages of our life.

This explosive convergence of demographic factors is therefore complex. It is necessary to not only implement new public policies at the transnational level in some cases but also promote the values of solidarity and intergenerational equity to ensure social cohesion and balance the rights of the present with those of future generations (Alkire and Jahan 2018). There should be a clear consideration of the benchmarks of intergenerational justice that are intended for society to ensure the financial sustainability of the welfare state. For example, regarding social security, both as an individual contributory endeavor and instantaneous solidarity between different generations, the rules must be clear, accountable, and in substantial harmony with the interests and preferences of the new generations.

The first challenge, which is a civilizational imperative, is to define and accept criteria of justice in both individual and collective choices (Rawls 1971). This challenge should be defined because the divergence of interests of different generations, which coexist with each other over extended periods of time, can give rise to a social equation that is difficult to solve. A new social contract that incorporates both intra- and intergenerational dimensions should be proposed and agreed on. Reinforcing the importance of solidarity bonds that unite generations is a collective aim that society must fully assume; therefore, it is important to guarantee the actual generations and net contributors to the functioning of the welfare state that their rights will be fully realized. The active and productive elements of society (of the younger generations) must therefore understand the importance of social cohesion, even in the face of necessary cost containment in social benefits. A fundamental issue is the financial sustainability of the social functions of the government; that is, the way in which we can presently guarantee to future generations that we are not mortgaging their future and that we can guarantee them a lifestyle in accordance with their expectations.

Then, we need to design a social contract that is not limited to the present generations but extends to the upcoming generations (Nunes et al. 2017). For the viability of this new social contract and under the assumption that there are limits to social solidarity even if compulsory, vigorous measures must be implemented to ensure that aging is associated with a good quality of life (Nussbaum 2009). One of the genetic landmarks of civilized countries is the existence of high levels of human development that will guarantee quality of life for all generations according to their age (Human Development Report 2016). Active, even positive, aging must be the cornerstone of the 21st-century society; it only makes sense to increase longevity if the quality of life remains stable (or even increases) over several generations (Nicholson et al. 2016). Increasing the levels of health literacy in the population is the central landmark of active aging along with an adequate inclusion of the senior population in society, namely promoting access to its recreational, social, or cultural activities. Empowering the elderly is an essential step toward a genuinely active aging policy. That is, full human development and corresponding social participation presuppose this ideal of intergenerational justice (Sen 1999).

As a collective responsibility of society, the state, third sector institutions, corporations, and social entrepreneurs, among other social agents, must decisively contribute to this objective. In addition, the family, which forms the core of human development, has the duty to bring about a possible balance between the individuation and the socialization of its members. Promoting ethical and social responsibility in providing the necessary support to the most vulnerable members, especially by utilizing the informal care that is frequently sought in an institutional environment nowadays, helps the community to become progressively age friendly. In short, active aging implies the implementation of the necessary structures for the creation of a *society for all ages*, promoting genuine solidarity between generations.

The inversion of the demographic pyramid that may occur due to a considerable increase in the average life expectancy of the population can lead to an increase in socially responsible citizens and consideration of new forms of active participation of pensioners to help mitigate the impact of the population's progressive aging on social security (The World Bank Group 2018). For example, the European Parliament approved a recommendation suggesting an increase in the average retirement age, albeit on a voluntary basis. This may also be considered as a career evolution in an inverted U in which after reaching the top, one may still be professionally useful, although in tasks where expertise and accumulated knowledge are paramount. Then, more exhaustive tasks – such as leadership – may be left to younger generations.

However, the modernization and sustainability of the welfare state also depend on a new fiscal policy that considers the reduction in birth rate and therefore, the need to reverse the current demographic trend. The financial flow to the welfare state can be only increased by broadening the tax base. This implies a fiscal policy that protects the incomes of families with descendants. Social benefits must be complemented by each citizen's individual responsibilities. In this context, the principle of subsidiarity assumes progressive importance and must be interpreted casuistically in the different manifestations of the welfare state. The co-responsibility of citizens who have the material conditions for this purpose should be regarded as an element to be considered for exercising responsible citizenship. Citizens must realize that they have rights and duties to themselves and their community. This implies a reformulation of the interrelation between the citizen and the state, especially in sectors in which individual (and household) responsibility is more easily demanded, such as higher education or health.

One of the most controversial issues is the discussion about welfare state financing models because it has a direct influence on people's quality of life. For example, one may ask if the traditional financing model based on taxes to a user/payer (co-payment) strategy should evolve (Khaleghian and Gupta 2005). However, this debate may give the impression that the scarcity of financial resources is the only problem regarding the viability of the welfare state. Indeed, if the wealth generated in a society does not grow more than expenditures, increasing the financing of a given social sector then implies making choices within a hierarchy of social priorities. Even in this soft version, critics say that the welfare state creates a *bottomless pit* and that the state is inexorably *hostage of the citizens* because the state is obliged to ensure access to all sorts of social benefits (Hoppe 2018).

This situation is aggravated by the recent sustained increase in the population's average life expectancy. To strike a balance between limited resources and social rights, economic policy must resort to the use of economic and financial instruments to fulfill the social functions of the government. That is, efficiency in resource allocation is a structural pillar of social policies. However, it must be stressed that efficiency is only a means to achieve an end. *Efficiency* should not be understood only as *saving* but rather as a tool that, at least in the first instance, contributes to equity. Therefore, it has an intrinsic ethical value in the modern welfare state.

A Modern Welfare State

In recent decades, the growing needs of the population have made it necessary to rethink the governance arrangements of the welfare state in all modern societies. In most countries, it is difficult to control the demographic transition associated with other factors, such as scientific and technological development (United Nations Population Fund 2008). Meanwhile, economic and cultural globalization via the redistribution of existing wealth worldwide has equalized the relative importance of different societies. Thus, a new reformist wave is needed to guarantee the core values of the welfare state without compromising its future viability.

The main public policy trend in many countries has been to ensure the sustainability of the welfare system through the implementation of structural measures that substantially change the relationship between the state and citizens, namely by redefining public policies to increase efficiency in resource allocation. Thus, an attempt should be made to determine the extent to which state failures in the provision of essential goods, such as waiting lists for surgery or poor educational performance, question the ability of public providers to effectively respond to citizens' preferences (Laugesen 2005). It can even be deduced that responsiveness should be a central element of a new ideological platform for the welfare state. In fact, state failures are particularly difficult to accept in modern societies because of the systematic scrutiny of different stakeholders (Boyne et al. 2003).

The redefinition of the state's core functions implies a modern and new approach to public management. In this context, Giandomenico Majone's proposal of a *regulatory state* was a welcomed solution in many countries (Majone 1997). Some of the strategies implemented to ensure the sustainability of the welfare state have been directed at reducing overall expenditure in this area and increasing financial transfers to the public systems. Sharing costs through the implementation of co-payments has also been a common practice in many developed countries, although limited to some extent. However, increasing the financial flows to a particular social area has a high opportunity cost because it implies the sacrifice of other essential goods. In other words, it involves making politically controversial choices about which social areas to select, namely health, education, social security, cultural activities, and/or research and development, among others. However, it is not only the high opportunity cost that is at stake; diverting resources from the private sector may compromise overall economic development.

The *regulatory state* is implemented through the functional split between the financing, the provision, and the regulation of the welfare state (Nunes et al. 2007). If the state needs to essentially ensure that all citizens have access to healthcare, education, or unemployment allowance, then the institutional nature of the provider is deemed irrelevant. This new conceptual paradigm considers that citizens must be able to satisfy their needs at the lowest possible cost (Boyer and Saillard 2002). Reinventing public administration means having this goal on the horizon. Then, the government does not have to be a *provider* in the strict sense of the term; rather, it should be the guarantor of citizens' access to essential goods and a supervisor of the system's functioning (Walshe 2003).

Substantially opening to the competitive market with different competing agents can be a source of efficiency and cost containment (Federowicz and Aguilera 2003). Meanwhile, the principle of freedom of consumer choice must be clearly assumed. Every citizen should be able to choose the service that best meets their needs and expectations. What is at stake is the development of a *government by contract*. This corresponds to the fragmentation of the administrative structure and replacement of the hierarchical structure (vertical and centralized) with new forms of coordination of activities based on contracts. It has been argued that contracting will increase accountability, reduce costs, and increase quality. This model is based on agency theory (principal/agent), in which the public/private organization provides a public service by delegation of the state. The establishment of contracts has been implemented in health, higher education, and even in the administration of justice (prisons) through the establishment of appropriate public/private partnerships (Sussex 2001).

Thus, a new public management system is necessary. The internal configuration of the welfare state must be reinvented to bring decision-makers closer to citizens and open the public sector to providers that best serve society's interests. In this way, the resources that citizens allocate to social goods will be better used, value for money will be increased, and inefficiency will be reduced to residual levels. However, in areas of strong social value, competition should not be seen as an end. The goal of a welfare state is not to generate profits; the aim is essentially to guarantee the basic rights of citizens, particularly when these rights are especially valued. The introduction of competitive market rules (which does not necessarily mean privatization) should therefore be seen as a tool for generating competitiveness and ensuring the economic sustainability of the system regarding the use of taxes. Thus, in the interface between private providers and the public sector, what is at stake is competition for the market (of public financing) and not competition within a single market, specific to each sector of activity.

No model can determine the *optimal weight* of social benefits. Studies argue that in many countries, the government is overburdened and that it is important to rethink the welfare state. The universality of public healthcare systems is a paradigmatic example (Tobin 2012). By using either principles or systematic imposition by international institutions (International Monetary Fund, World Bank) to control the public deficit, the problem of financing a welfare state is perhaps one of the most controversial because it is a serious issue with direct influence on the quality of citizens' life (Nunes and Rego 2014). If the wealth generated by the economy does not grow more than the expenditures in the next years, increasing the financing of the welfare state then implies making choices within the framework of a hierarchy of social priorities. However, new public management may not be enough to make the welfare state viable; then, direct citizen participation can become a necessity. Importantly, transitioning from a tax-based financing model to a mixed model based on taxes and co-payments (user/payer) requires a reduction in the tax burden. At the conceptual level, the principle of the social division of responsibility allows for the implementation of a co-payment strategy.

Assume that all citizens in a modern society must have equal opportunity to access certain social goods, such as education or health. Then within the limits of its economic and financial resources, the state must guarantee such access, particularly when it comes to meeting citizens' basic needs. Note that there are significant differences between different social goods. If we take education as an example, the state will always be responsible for ensuring high levels of coverage in terms of compulsory education. At this level, any kind of direct co-payment of citizens or their families in the public system, regardless of the level of household income, seems unreasonable. In higher education, the partial introduction of co-payments may be legitimate. In fact, regardless of whether there is a support system for the worse-off students (so that they are not unfairly discriminated against in accessing higher education), this level of education confers not only a social advantage but also a higher average level of income. This must be considered, at least in part, as an investment of the household in the education of their offspring.

This perspective requires that the core values of modern societies should be ensured without compromising the necessary efficiency in resource allocation (Breyer 1982). It is a new vision for public administration and for the complex interrelationships between the government and other sectors of the economy (Mallin 2018). Rethinking the welfare state implies rebuilding its internal architecture by considering economic and cultural globalization, and the revolution generated by both the society of knowledge and the digital transformation (Ireland-Piper and Wolff 2017).

Conclusion

The welfare state that has been built over the past decades in many modern countries must be considered an important civilizational achievement, allowing the general population to reach satisfactory levels of well-being (Macklin 2012). Still, we have not been able to completely eradicate social exclusion due to its significantly associated poverty rate, even in societies with greater human development. In fact, people with disabilities, dependent elderly people, single parents, homeless, low-paid workers, or prisoners are particularly vulnerable groups whose poverty is generally associated with the phenomenon of social exclusion. Thus, a modern welfare state must have a clear perception of the phenomenon of poverty because it has serious consequences for well-being and for individuals' achievements in life. For instance, according to Eurostat, 18% of the European population still experiences income poverty (Eurostat 2019). Indeed, poverty is a multidimensional problem that needs to be addressed (Alkire and Foster 2011). Child-specific deprivation is even more problematic, and monetary child poverty and material deprivation should be a priority of the welfare state (Chzhen et al. 2016), with huge repercussions on health.

However, the welfare state must be essentially reinvented at the level of financial sustainability. Despite the implementation of measures to increase efficiency, a welfare state's economic and financial viability has not been guaranteed yet. The welfare state should be modern and sustainable. It must respect the core values of modern societies and not forget the impact of economic and cultural globalization on citizens' income levels and well-being. However, economic development must not be dissociated from a concrete model of human development. As one of its core objectives, the welfare state must promote the development of society considering not only traditional development indicators but also complementary indicators, such as the Multidimensional Poverty Index (MPI), the Gender Inequality Index (GII), or even the Inequality-Adjusted Human Development Index (IHDI) (Alkire and Foster 2010). A modern and sustainable vision of the welfare state may be the answer to a variable geometry that exists on a global scale.

References

Alkire S and Foster J. 2010. Designing the inequality-adjusted human development index. *Human Development Research Paper*: 28.

Alkire S and Foster J. 2011. Counting and multidimensional poverty measurement. *Journal of Public Economics* 95 (7): 476–487.

Alkire S and Jahan S. 2018. The new global MPI 2018: Aligning with the sustainable development goals. HDRO Occasional Paper, United Nations Development Programme (UNDP), New York.

Boyer R and Saillard Y. 2002. *Regulation theory. The state of the art*. Routledge, London.

Boyne G, Farrell C, Law J et al. 2003. *Evaluating public management reforms*. Open University Press, Buckingham.

Breyer S. 1982. *Regulation and its reform*. Harvard University Press, Cambridge.

Callahan D and Gaylin W. 2017. How long a life is enough life? *The Hastings Center Report* 47 (4): 16–18.

Choices in Health Care. 1992. *A report by the government committee on choices in health care*, Choices in Health Care, The Netherlands.

Chzhen Y, de Neubourg C, Plavgo I et al. 2016. Child poverty in the European Union: The multiple overlapping deprivation analysis approach (EU-MODA). *Child Indicators Research* 9: 335–356. https://doi.org/10.1007/s12187-015-9321-7.

Daniels N and Sabin J. 2002. *Setting limits fairly*. Oxford University Press, New York.

Dworkin R. 2000. *Sovereign virtue. The theory and practice of equality*. Harvard University Press, Cambridge.

European Commission. 2017. *The 2018 Ageing Report, underlying assumptions & projection methodologies*. European Commission, Luxembourg.

European Commission. 2019. Gender equality strategy. Achievements and key areas for action. https://ec.europa.eu/info/policies/justice-and-fundamental-rights/gender-equality/gender-equality-strategy_en [Accessed 12 January 2021].

Eurostat. 2019. Archive: Income poverty statistics. *Eurostat Statistics Explained*. https://ec.europa.eu/eurostat/statistics-explained/index.php?title=Income_poverty_statistics&oldid=440992 [Accessed 02 June 2021].

Federowicz A and Aguilera R. 2003. *Corporate governance in a changing economic and political environment: Trajectories of institutional change*. Palgrave Macmillan, New York.

Hayek FA. 1976. *Law, legislation and liberty. Volume 2. The mirage of social justice*. Routledge & Kegan Paul, London and Henley.

Hoppe HH. 2018. *Social democracy*. Mises Institute, Auburn.

Human Development Report 2016. 2016. *Human development for everyone*. United Nations Development Programme, New York.

Ireland-Piper D and Wolff L. 2017. *Global governance and regulation. Order and disorder in the 21st century*. Routledge, London.

Khaleghian P and Gupta M. 2005. Public management and the essential public health functions, *World Development* 33 (7): 1083–1099.

Kumar V and Sundarraj R. 2018. *Global innovation and economic value*. Springer, New Delhi.

Laugesen M. 2005. Why some market reforms lack legitimacy in health care. *Journal of Health Politics, Policy & Law* 30 (6): 1065–1100.

Macklin R. 2012. *Ethics in global health: Research, policy, and practice*. Oxford University Press, New York.

Majone G. 1997. From the positive to the regulatory state. *Journal of Public Policy* 17 (2): 139–167.

Mallin C. 2018. *Corporate governance*. Oxford University Press, Oxford, 6th edition.

McLuhan M and Powers B. 1989. *Chapter 1: The resonating interval in the global village. Transformations in world life and media in the 21st century*. Oxford University Press, Oxford.

Nagel T. 1991. *Equality and partiality*. Oxford University Press, New York.

Nicholson T, Admay C, Shakow A et al. 2016. Double standards in global health: Medicine, human rights law and multidrug-resistant TB treatment policy. *Health and Human Rights* 18 (1): 85–102.

Nozick R. 1974. *Anarchy, state and utopia*. Basic Books, New York.

Nunes C. 2013. *€uro=Neoliberalismo + Socialismo*. Vida Económica, Porto.

Nunes R. 2020. Addressing gender inequality to promote basic human rights and development: A global perspective. *CEDIS Working Papers* 2020 (1). http://cedis.fd.unl.pt/blog/project/addressing-gender-inequality-to-promote-basic-human-rights-and-development-a-global-perspective/.

Nunes R, Brandão C and Rego G. 2011. Public accountability and sunshine healthcare regulation. *Health Care Analysis* 19 (4): 352–364.

Nunes R, Nunes SB and Rego G. 2017. Healthcare as a universal right. *Journal of Public Health* 25: 1–9.

Nunes R and Rego G. 2014. Priority setting in health care: A complementary approach. *Health Care Analysis* 22 (3): 2, 92–303.

Nunes R, Rego G and Brandão C. 2007. The rise of independent regulation in health care. *Health Care Analysis* 15 (3): 169–177.

Nussbaum M. 2009. Creating capabilities – The human development approach and its implementation. *Hyparia* 24 (3): 211–215.

Olshansky SJ, Martin GM and Kirkland JL. 2015. *The longevity dividend*. Cold Spring Harbor Laboratory Press, Cold Spring Harbor, New York.

Power M. 1997. *The audit society: Rituals of verification*. Oxford University Press, Oxford.

Rawls J. 1971. *A theory of justice*. Harvard University Press, New York.

Samuelson P and Nordhaus W. 2009. *Economics*. McGraw-Hill Irwin, Boston, 19th edition.

Sen A. 1999. *Development as freedom*. Knopf, New York.

Sussex J. 2001. *The economics of the private finance initiative in the NHS*. Office of Health Economics, London.

Tobin J. 2012. *The right to health in international law*. Oxford University Press, Oxford.

United Nations Population Fund. 2008. *State of world population 2008*. Reaching Common Ground: Culture, Gender and Human Rights, New York.

Vasak K. 1977. A 30 year struggle. The sustained efforts to give force of law to the Universal Declaration of Human Rights. *UNESCO Courier*, November, pp. 29–32. https://unesdoc.unesco.org/ark:/48223/pf0000048063 [Accessed 15 January 2021].

von Mises L. 2007. *Human action: A treatise on economics*. Liberty Fund Edition, Indianapolis.

Walshe K. 2003. *Regulating healthcare. A prescription for improvement?* State of Health Series. Open University Press, Maidenhead.

The World Bank. 2016. Development goals in an era of demographic change. Global Monitoring Report 2015/2016, Washington, DC. DOI: 10.1596/978-1-4648-0669-8.

The World Bank Group. 2018. *Implementing the 2030 agenda*. 2018 Update, Washington, DC.

3   A Universal Right to Healthcare of Variable Geometry[1]

Most developed societies recognize the existence of a basic right to healthcare access and consider it a positive welfare right (Daniels 1998). It can even be one of the most important achievements of pluralistic and secular societies, rather, even a civilization-based right. This right can be an expression of human dignity. In Europe, Art. 3 of the Convention on Human Rights and Biomedicine (Council of Europe 1996) implicitly recognizes the existence of a right to healthcare access, even if limited by economic constraints. This article states that "Parties, taking into account health needs and available resources, shall take appropriate measures with a view to providing, within their jurisdiction, equitable access to healthcare of appropriate quality."

The right to healthcare access is crucial to the pursuit of an effective equality of opportunity in a free and inclusive society. Diseases, deficiencies, and disabilities restrict the opportunities that otherwise would be within an individual's reach. These are unfair situations and not just the result of random forces of nature. That is, all citizens should have the necessary resources for an acceptable physical and psychological performance. This can enable them to access a reasonable and appropriate range of social goods (Daniels 1985).

In modern countries, one of the visions of distributive justice that is in accordance with the conceptual formulation of the welfare state is perhaps John Rawls' (1971) egalitarian theory. This theory rests on the concept of social contract. Based on this contract, a democratic and pluralistic society that is properly organized and structured has fundamental values of individual freedom and equal access to primary social goods. Therefore, the principle of equal opportunity becomes the main instrument that determines the social, educational, and health policies in most advanced democracies. The existence of institutions legitimized by democratic power emanates from this model of social organization. For Rawls, this is a prerequisite to the widespread implementation of these values. However, utilitarian values should also be considered, such as the necessary cost containment in healthcare, and cost-benefit, cost-utility, and cost-effectiveness analysis.

The right to healthcare access should be interpreted considering egalitarian theories, including the precept of fair equality of opportunity. That is, every citizen should start their social life with similar circumstances in biological and social levels so that they can develop their talents and capabilities in accordance with

DOI: 10.4324/9781003241065-4

the principle of individual freedom. Moreover, this institutional transcendentalism may be a means for an overarching goal of a full human development. According to Amartya Sen (1989, 1999), capabilities expansion is essential for true enjoyment of freedom.

The main objective of this chapter is to suggest a conceptual foundation for a universal right to healthcare access that implies that all humankind should be enabled to access healthcare of appropriate quality. This universal human right is a moral right that can also become a legal right. A second objective is to propose the necessary tools so that access to healthcare of appropriate quality is viable in a specific commonwealth in accordance with available resources. This architecture of principles is not intended to suggest that everyone in the world is entitled to every health service available or that everyone is entitled to the same health status. This status depends on many different circumstances such as the familial, social, and economic conjuncture of the specific person and community. Moreover, I do not intend to suggest that such a framework can prioritize healthcare access over other important goods, although a similar reasoning can be applied with this goal.

Ethical Background

Healthcare access can be a right of citizens and communities that should be implemented through the joint responsibility of both. Each state should promote and ensure healthcare access to all citizens within the human, technical, and financial limits (Abel-Smith 1994). It is also a responsibility of the international community: international law tackles a range of issues such as access to medicines in low-income countries (Tobin 2012).

However, healthcare must compete with other social goods. Thus, resources should be used for treatments with proven effectiveness and with the least possible waste. That is, the implementation of a universal human right to healthcare access should be based on the following structuring principles:

1   Equal opportunity,
2   solidarity,
3   evidence-based practice, and
4   efficiency in resource allocation.

Thus, the first principle refers to the need to ensure equal access to healthcare of appropriate quality, overcoming at least some of the existing financial and non-financial barriers (Daniels and Sabin 2002). A concrete application of the principle of equal opportunity is the idea that no citizen should be excluded from the health system due to a lack of resources. Indeed, most developed societies claim the premise that all citizens should have access to the health system. To achieve a balance between the right of access to healthcare and the shortage of resources, it seems to be essential to define *appropriate quality*. This definition, in turn, will politically condition the constitution of a basic package of healthcare (a decent minimum in the philosophical perspective). The reasonableness criterion must preponderate, that is, what the *reasonable* citizen may choose given the circumstances (Williams et al. 2012).

The second principle aims to ensure that the way in which the basic ring of healthcare services is financed in a tired system ensures the principle of equity in access. From the perspective of equal opportunity, the economic and financial instruments that ensure the fulfillment of this principle are not particularly relevant. The financing model of the health system can be even less important. Public systems can be based on taxes, such as in the UK (Beveridge-type systems), on a compulsory public insurance according to the income of the citizens, such as in the Netherlands or Germany (Bismarck-type systems), or on both schemes, such as in mixed systems. The goals include equal opportunity in access to healthcare of acceptable quality and geographical/spatial equity. In the past decades, there has been controversy over the strengths and weaknesses of Beveridge- compared to Bismarck-type public integrated systems. Each system must be adapted to the specificities of a particular culture (Veeder and Peebles-Wilkins 2001). However, equitable funding presupposes some form of social solidarity. "Solidarity is the awareness of unity and a willingness to bear the consequences of it. Unity indicates the presence of a group of people with a common history and common convictions and ideals" (Choices in Healthcare 1992). Solidarity can be voluntary, as when people behave out of humanistic motives, or compulsory, as when the government taxes the population to provide services to all. The financing of public health systems is already clearly progressive through direct and indirect taxes charged to taxpayers. However, another issue relates to the possibility of introducing co-payments for services (consultation, surgery, or diagnosis). Here, the co-payment may have two distinct purposes:

1   It provides discipline and rationalizes the demand for healthcare.
2   It can also help finance the system.

While there is no objection to the implementation of the principle of co-payments, the tax burden is relatively high in many countries. Thus, it may be socially unjust to double citizens' taxes (co-payment and taxes); therefore, this measurement might jeopardize the social perception of the need for a public healthcare system (moral skimming). Moreover, co-payments in the public system may originate professional skimming, and therefore, patient skimming. Indeed, both high-quality professionals, such as middle-class patients, can flow to the private sector due to the expected adjustment of private players to the introduction of co-payments in the public service. The problem of health system financing is one of the most burning issues of controversy because it is a serious matter that directly influences the quality of life of all people. However, introducing the discussion around financing models, that is, if the traditional model of tax-based financing should evolve into a dynamic of user/payer, can give the impression that the only problem of the welfare state is the shortage of financial resources (Wall and Owen 1999).

Further, there are clear political limits with the principle of progressive taxation as one of the core criteria for the funding of the health system and as a means to achieve fairness. These limits are imposed for two reasons. First, the principle established by Arthur Laffer in 1980 reaffirms the conviction that there is both direct and indirect tax evasion as well as other tax liabilities if the tax limits are unreasonable. Excessive progressivity will lead to a perverse and counterproductive effect because the taxpayer will perceive the taxes to be excessive. Therefore, the total amount of resources may be considerably reduced. Second, Rawls' difference principle suggests the existence of private property (substantially affected if taxes are exaggerated) that is an essential tool to generate wealth in a fair and democratic society; this achieves the goal of protecting the disadvantaged.

The following criterion refers to a clear determination of the effectiveness of most diagnosis and treatment modalities in health, that is, the acceptance of scientific evidence as an operational criterion. Evidence-based medicine (EBM) is the paradigm of this quiet revolution in clinical practice. The most common definition of EBM is taken from David Sackett: EBM is "the conscientious, explicit and judicious use of current best evidence in making decisions about the care of the individual patient. It means integrating individual clinical expertise with the best available external clinical evidence from systematic research" (Sackett 2000). This concept should be seen as a valuable tool for physicians and patients. A stronger level of evidence leads to a greater degree of clinical recommendation.

This definition is part of the dynamics of the doctor–patient relationship, that is, a constant search for the best interest of the patient and their quality of life via a dynamic perspective of medical practice (Leathard 2000). In fact, doctors and patients have never previously had access to so much information about healthcare. Unfortunately, much of this information is confusing or is biased and/ or fragmented. For the clinician, it can be particularly difficult to discern which information is based on the latest scientific evidence. EBM aims to provide the best evidence for physicians and patients to jointly adopt the best course of action.

To achieve this goal, critical evaluations of evidence that originate from systematic reviews of the literature must be conducted. This can lead to practical guidelines in conjunction with local circumstances. These clinical guidelines should always be integrated with individual patient information; they can be only considered mandatory when a compulsory feature cannot distort the essence of the doctor–patient relationship. Rather, the guidelines should help clinicians make the most efficient and effective decision. Nonvalidated therapies and even harmful traditional practices should also be evaluated by EBM.

These critical reviews of the evidence take the form of meta-analyses and mega-meta-analyses in which specialized centers coordinate at a global level (e.g., Cochrane) to statistically evaluate the results of several published studies on specific topics. Thus, this process can extract what seems to be the best possible evidence on the effectiveness of a particular treatment or intervention. This methodology currently has been used mostly with pharmaceuticals but can be also applied in any field of health.

EBM can also serve as a tool for resource allocation. That is, the economic and financial constraints, and the objective application of distributive justice criteria require that the scarce resources allocated to health be used in clinical treatments with proven effectiveness. The global production and distribution of pharmaceuticals fuel this perspective (Deloitte 2011; Sahu 2014). If a treatment has no proven clinical effectiveness, then it is not ethically legitimate to use it because there is no valid reason to include it in the basic healthcare provision. EBM has another aspect: it can prioritize healthcare based on effectiveness. However, the implementation of criteria for clinical effectiveness does not object, in principle, to the restriction of innovative and expensive treatments, provided that this decision is transparent and shared with society via democratic and consensual procedures. Thus, EBM has a double objective: to assist clinical practice and to restrict treatments with unproven effectiveness according to the criteria of distributive justice. It is increasingly seen as an essential tool for the provision of a reasonable healthcare level and to ensure fair access to the system (Wiseman et al. 2003).

However, equal opportunity, solidarity, and evidence-based practice should be in accordance with efficient use of resources. Here, efficiency is considered as an ethical imperative. This should be a structural pillar of health policy. In the health sector, economic rationality should be used to guarantee the right of access to healthcare of appropriate quality. Thus, market and free competition in health must have this basic right of the citizens as a prerequisite. However, efficiency and equal opportunity have opposite signs after a certain time; thus, political decisions are needed to balance the interests at stake and decide according to the prevailing social values. For example, waiting lists in healthcare are open and do not limit the demand for healthcare, improve efficiency, and combat waste. However, an efficient healthcare system reduces waiting time to a socially acceptable minimum. Pursuing economic efficiency may eliminate some types of treatment from the health system only when the waste is null (Kapiriri et al. 2007). Thus, efficiency in resource allocation is an ethical imperative that society must fully assume.

Another example is the use of generic drugs, based on the assumption (not always valid) that this type of medicine has the lowest price in the market. This practice can safeguard the principle of freedom of prescription and not jeopardize the best interests of the patient. Generic drugs should not be considered an option but rather a professional duty. The presumable savings via the use of generics can channel resources to other areas of health (e.g., orphan drugs). This can improve the overall performance of the system (Rego et al. 2002). Indeed, the high opportunity cost in most clinical choices as well as the limits of available resources determine that any decision in healthcare that has financial and budgetary impact should be carefully evaluated insofar as the rights of other patients are put into question (even statistic patients).

On the basis of these criteria, I suggest the existence of a universal right to healthcare as a basic right of humankind. Basic because it is inherent to the equal dignity of every person. Universal implies that everyone in every country should have access to healthcare of appropriate quality. Although this is an acknowledged human right and there is a robust relationship between health and broad social arrangements, problems remain. As suggested by Sridhar Venkatapuram (2009), even if every human being has a moral entitlement to a capability to be healthy, how can this right be enjoyed in countries with different levels of development?

Should low-income countries still depend on international charity, of rich countries good will, as happens with COVID-19 vaccination? Or should we suggest a realistic and rather, an achievable way to implement universal coverage? Indeed, I believe that the concept of *appropriate quality* is context specific and resource driven because the world is not uniformly developed. Adjusting the right to healthcare access to the available resources (determined by each country's political process) is the challenge suggested in the next section.

Strengths and Limits of a Universal Right to Healthcare Access

Within the framework of the principles highlighted in the previous section, the existence of a universal right to healthcare access of appropriate quality is based on the premise that in any commonwealth, any person is entitled to this moral right although its specific legal operationalization may differ in societies with different levels of development (Nunes et al. 2017). As stated in a 2012 editorial in *The Lancet*, "The vision of universal health coverage is rapidly becoming a reality, with access to healthcare no longer the privilege of a few, but the birth right of many" (The Lancet 2012). Persad and Emanuel (2017) suggest that the goal of universal health coverage should be a global one with three fundamental values that support this proposal: utility, equity, and priority to the worst off. Norman Daniels also agrees that healthcare access is a human right of special moral importance because it contributes to the range of opportunities open to all of us. However, while Daniels suggests the need for *fair processes* to deliver healthcare in any given society, they do not suggest a substantive approach to the citizens' entitlements (Daniels 2008). Jonathan Wolff departs from cautious idealism suggesting that the implementation of the right to healthcare is a duty of the government. However, on the basis of international declarations and conventions, the author makes a move toward the responsibility of the international community, claiming that rich countries have a moral duty to assist low-income countries because healthcare is, in this perspective, an enforceable claim (Wolff 2012). On the basis of the Brazilian experience, Octávio Ferraz (2020) refers to the judicialization of healthcare as a tool for this right to be enjoyed by everyone. But should this be the proper way societies deal with the delivery of healthcare? Is it acceptable that the constitution, or any other legal arrangement, refers to a level of provision that society simply has not the means to comply with?

In this chapter, I will argue that the existence of a universal right to healthcare access goes beyond a universal health coverage *stricto sensu*. This is because accepting healthcare access as a basic humanitarian right implies that the basic package is progressively adjusted to the available resources of a particular society. It is adjusted as an ethical imperative and not only as a social or political compromise, as universal coverage seems to imply.

Meanwhile, it is important to determine how to promote this right at a global level, considering the absence of true universal enforcement institutions and of global governance arrangements (Brock 2009; Ireland-Piper and Wolff 2017). The existence of this universal right is part of a global perspective of justice, as suggested by Amartya Sen in the sense of a global social choice (Sen 2009). This argument emphasizes that the principle of equal opportunity must be of transnational application, ensuring harmonious development of all people and all communities (Sen 1989, 1999). Indeed, in the absence of global sovereign state/global sovereign institutions, what sort of international reforms can be implemented to make the world less unjust? John Rawls (1971) and other supporters of the social contract theory relate distributive justice to the existence of sovereignty and fair institutions. In other words, they argue that only a sovereign state can apply a concept of justice by resorting to a perfect set of just and transcendental institutions.

This chapter claims that it is possible to reconcile the right to self-determination with the ideal of a *minimal humanitarianism* despite the lack of a perfectly fair global society. This *minimal humanitarianism* applies to a set of social goods such as education, shelter, and food. However, there is no doubt that health is among the most fundamental social goods. Therefore, it is possible to consider the right to healthcare access as a basic and universal right, even if distinct communities have different rates of development and diverse resource availability. This reality should not prevent the international community from establishing spatial equity as an ideal, that is, any person in the world should have access to healthcare of appropriate quality.

The Human Development Index clearly shows the variable geometry in development across different countries and communities (Human Development Report 2020). Variable geometry describes the idea of a method of differentiated integration of countries worldwide that acknowledges that there are important, even irreconcilable, differences within the political, economic, social, and cultural structure of different countries. Therefore, it allows for different levels of access to healthcare and for different interpretations of healthcare of appropriate quality but always in accordance with the United Nations' (UN's) concept of a decent standard of living.

For instance, recognizing this variable geometry, the Treaty of Lisbon, which is a legal instrument that seeks to establish a charter of fundamental rights of all citizens of the European family, reflects the need to harmonize different cultures and social development models so that the collective future of the peoples of the European Union crosses smoothly (Treaty of Lisbon 2007). In Article 168, this treaty acknowledges that the

> Union action shall respect the responsibilities of the Member States for the definition of their health policy and for the organization and delivery of health services and medical care. The responsibilities of the Member States shall include the management of health services and medical care as well as the allocation of the resources assigned to them.

Following this European experience, a universal right to healthcare access of appropriate quality can be proposed worldwide if its limits are objectively accepted in accordance with the level of development of each specific country (Pogge 2008).

The question to ask is, "what medical care and health services should integrate the healthcare system?" In this regard, Daniels et al. (1996) make a clear distinction between preferences (amenities) and needs (fundamental) concerning health. These are based on the distinction between preferences and needs, as described in the famous Dutch report on health priorities, Choices in Healthcare (1992). This report suggested certain orthodontic treatments with a purely aesthetic purpose be excluded from the basic system as well as certain psychotherapeutic interventions (counseling) that seek only to improve comfort and quality of life. According to this report, even some infertility treatments (human-assisted procreation and repro-genetics) may be excluded from the basic healthcare package because they were not considered essential for a *normal* social functioning.

That is, based on the assumption that resources are limited and the cost of healthcare tends to grow exponentially, a fair society must establish, in accordance with predefined and mutually agreed rules, methods of inclusion and exclusion of certain basic package interventions (Gallego et al. 2011; Gibson et al. 2002). Indeed, rationing in health is essentially due to the increase in population's average life expectancy, the increase in consumption of healthcare, and unprecedented development in medicine including new pharmaceuticals such as pharmacogenomics (Teagarden et al. 2003). I agree with Norman Daniels and James Sabin (Daniels and Sabin 1997, 1998), who stated that rationing of scarce goods must be performed according to the principle of public accountability (Friedman 2008). This is because it is inevitable to set priorities in healthcare. That is, society should be informed about the criteria that guided these decisions by resorting to appropriate, fair, and transparent procedures (Daniels et al. 2003). This implies the presence of a specific set of conditions, including the framework that Daniels and Sabin designated, for accountability and reasonableness: publicity condition, relevance condition, revision and appeals condition, and regulative condition.

To find the balance between an existing variable geometry and the actual level of resources of each specific commonwealth, one can find compatibility between Daniels' accountability for reasonableness and the World Health Organization's integrated view of health. Indeed, I propose an evolution of Daniels' account of justice in healthcare access because their *normal* functioning criterion as a standard for prioritizing is changed by a more flexible, responsive, and adjustable *needs* criterion. The perspective of justice as fairness implies that any citizen should have access to a decent minimum regarding healthcare, education, and other social goods, therefore guaranteeing a decent standard of living.

However, the guarantee of an effective opportunity to everyone should be reevaluated in light of available resources and the need to allocate them efficiently to different social goods. I suggest the implementation of a mathematical function that can be represented graphically in the form of an equal opportunity function, (EO)F, as in Figure 3.1 (Nunes and Rego 2014).

This function is suggested to promote an ethical reasoning that can support a framework for establishing priorities in healthcare within a specific community that involves a convergence between the concepts of vertical and horizontal

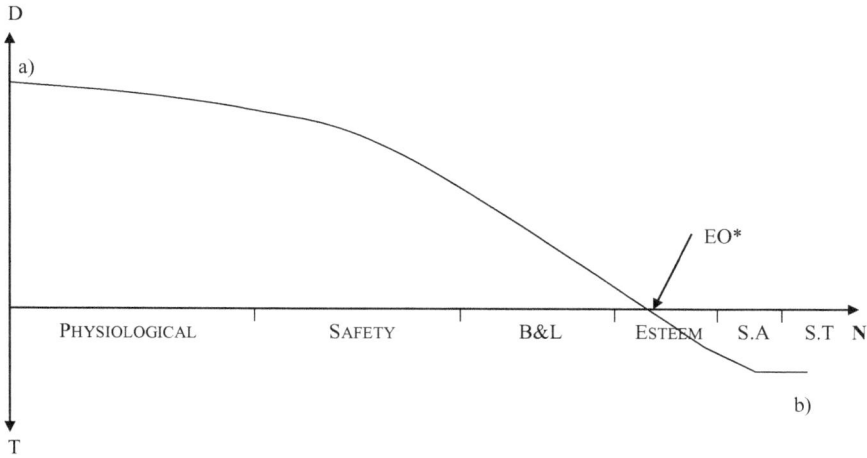

LEGEND:

D: Healthcare Delivery
T: Tiering
N: Needs (Maslow)
B&L: Belongingness and Love
S.A: Self-Actualization
S.T: Self-Transcendence
EO*: Point EO (point equal opportunity)

Figure 3.1 Equal Opportunity Function (EO)F.

equity. The (EO)F suggests a theoretical approach that reconciles the way equals should be treated equally and unequals, unequally. Two variables seem paramount for an accurate graphic representation of (EO)F:

1   X-axis represents the variable *hierarchy of needs*. The well-known Maslow needs are displayed in a progressive line including physiological, safety, belongingness and love, esteem, self-actualization, and self-transcendence.
2   Y-axis shapes the variable *type* and *level* of access to healthcare. The maximum value of this variable is represented by the universality and comprehensiveness of the public services. The minimum value below the X-axis is left to the individual responsibility and not to the public beneficence.

In this perspective, healthcare delivery has two main components clearly separated by a specific moment: point EO* in the (EO)F. On the upper side of the Y-axis, the financial burden of the system is publicly supported by the taxpayer. On the lower side, a mix between the *needs* criteria (i.e., the lower-level needs) and the financial constraints of the healthcare system implicate a personal, not societal, level of commitment to one's own health. Therefore, the public provision of healthcare is no longer mandatory. Most healthcare systems in developed countries are segmented, with at least two tiers. Further, alternative coverage schemes do exist, including private health insurance or out-of-pocket payments. This point EO* can vary depending on different variables, namely citizen's democratic choices. However, it can be situated schematically in the graphic area corresponding to what Maslow defined as esteem needs.

Ideally, with no resource constraints, all citizens may have access to all healthcare services and to every kind of innovation in medicine. However, as described by Penelope Mullen and Peter Spurgeon "the demand for healthcare is infinite and so rationing is inevitable"; thus, the conceptual paradigm of health policies all over the world is making explicit or implicit choices (Mullen and Spurgeon 2000). Indeed, all societies face the problem of choosing between competitive social goods; moreover, this trend is not slowing down. On the contrary, it is not possible, even in rich countries, to satisfy all the (Maslow) esteem and self-actualization needs nor all the individual preferences in healthcare. From an ethical perspective, this framework allows one to conceptualize a fair way to establish priorities in healthcare, and even establish priorities between healthcare and other social goods.

The combination of Daniels' accountability for reasonableness, that is, the publicity, relevance, revision, appeals and regulative conditions, with the (EO)F can allow a specific commonwealth to determine the cutoff line between healthcare provision and personal responsibility in a fair and transparent way. The suggested framework can distinguish between high and low degree needs, for example, a heart attack or a back pain, though they may need differential treatment. The (EO)F will determine, in advance, if the treatment needed is or is not in the basic package. Afterward, the application of Daniels' framework will validate this choice in a publicly accountable way. This methodology can also enable the decision-maker to choose between alternative treatments, although with very different costs. For instance, while selecting a pacemaker, both the predicted clinical outcomes and the costs involved should be considered.

This model is also applicable in societies with very different levels of development, including both advanced democracies and developing countries. This perspective is also compatible with other axiological references such as the capacity to function or achieve a minimally decent life (Shue 1980; Held 1995; Nussbaum 2009; Venkatapuram 2011). The balance between the social goods that people may or may not be entitled to should be preferably reached through democratic arrangements, but always in accordance with a socioeconomically determined decision-making process. In less developed societies and in direct accordance with the availability of resources, a progressive slide away from the maximalist curve may occur in accordance with the vertical equity principle (Figure 3.2). Nevertheless, higher grade needs should always prevail over lower healthcare needs.

The concrete application of the EO(F) should consider accountability for reasonableness (Hasman and Holm 2005; Jansson 2007; Rid 2009; Syrett 2008). It means that publicity, relevance, revision, appeals, and regulative conditions

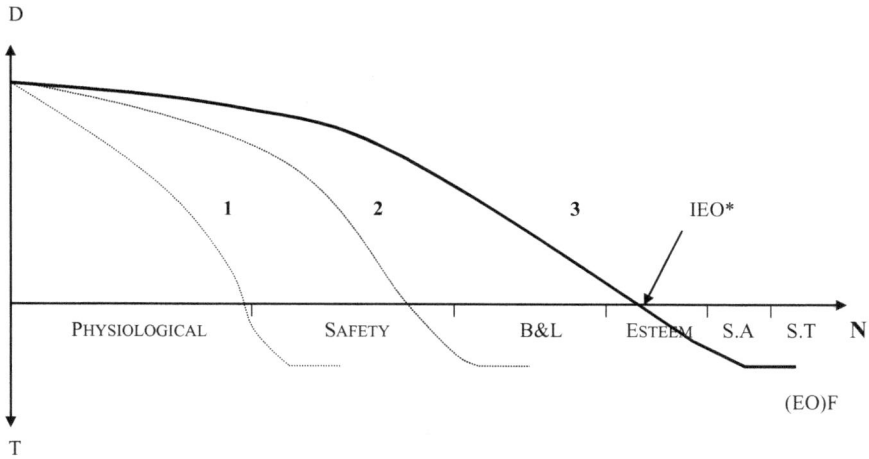

LEGEND:

1: Effective sub-maximalist curve: Slide away from maximalist curve for drastic economic and social reasons, for example, underdeveloped societies that score very low in the Human Development Index.

2: Effective sub-maximalist curve: Slide away from maximalist curve for moderate economic and social reasons, for example, societies with a moderate score in the Human Development Index.

3: Maximalist Curve: Expected equal opportunity function (EO)F in developed countries and modern democracies.

Figure 3.2 Equal Opportunity Function (EO)F – Variable Geometry.

should be applied by each commonwealth to determine the exact EO* point, that is, the concrete level of healthcare available to each citizen. However, I emphasize that the societal duties of health promotion are also underwritten by the principle of beneficence (Kelleher 2014). Both individual and public beneficence should be reflected in any society's health policy. Any political community is under a justice-based obligation of specific beneficence toward their members. According to Meier and Gostin (2018), both global institutions for public health and international law are fundamental for a global health governance. Further, the existence of a multi-sectoral array of global organizations in health and healthcare delivery is an important driver of change (Gostin and Meier 2020). However, international bureaucracies and conflicting interest frequently prevent the evolving relationship between human rights, global governance, and public health.

At a global level, if all human societies are regarded as a large political community, then efforts should be made so that these values are universally shared and the correlative rights are universally enjoyed. The fact that hundreds of millions of people on this planet do not have access to healthcare of appropriate quality does not preclude the proposal of realistic ways of approaching this dramatic problem.

The virtue of the (EO)F strategy, namely the possibility that there is a progressive slide away of the curve adjusting the deliverance to the existing resources, is that it can be applied in any country, regardless of the level of development and without interfering with the right of self-determination of that specific community. Indeed, it is the progressive implementation of a social structure that enables citizens to enjoy basic rights that can promote a different evolution in the world's future order. Civilized countries should promote these values sustainably so that every country will be compelled to implement a public healthcare system, although with different rhythms.

In underdeveloped countries, this perspective can be the starting point for the construction of a public healthcare system that will steadily develop in accordance with available resources in a fair and publicly accountable way. Moreover, such a transparent system can be internationally monitored. Thus, external resources can be more easily conveyed via the social responsibility of developed countries or even transnational corporations. The example of COVAX (COVID-19 Vaccines Global Access) as an international initiative to promote equitable access to vaccination, including partners such as coalition for epidemic preparedness innovations (CEPI), the vaccine alliance (GAVI) the world health organization (WHO), or UN Children's Fund (UNICEF), is an example that international support for global health will always be welcomed and is compatible with this perspective. Further, low- and middle-income countries, and even failed states (collapsed, with high levels of conflict, dangerous and disputed by rival factions) can be enrolled in this evolution. Indeed, promoting healthcare access in failed states will be an important step to protect their citizens, neighboring states, and the global community due to the difficulty in border control (Rotberg 2003).

This ethical framework suggests that the moral and legal concept of a universal right of access to healthcare of appropriate quality may be indexed to the level of economic development in a particular community. Therefore, different degrees of healthcare provision are still compatible with a universal dimension of this right. It is true that the quality of the health systems in developed countries depends largely on their economic power. However, this assumption does not preclude the possibility of a progressive implementation of a healthcare system in accordance with the financial constraints of each particular community. Moreover, the steady development of such a system may be an example of societal transformation that is well received by developed countries; in turn, this can further stimulate willingness to contribute to such an endeavor.

One should bear in mind that it is not possible to unilaterally change the world's order. Nor is it possible, or desirable, to surpass the long-standing right of self-determination of all countries and their sovereignty. Therefore, developed countries have an ethical obligation to fairly distribute the vast resources at their disposal in a pragmatic and realistic way. Although not ideal, this framework has at least the potential to provide healthcare of appropriate quality to all people in the world. Thus, far from legitimating the existing inequalities at a worldwide level, this approach appeals for a true global change in income distribution. The practical implementation of the right to healthcare can even contribute to the reduction of poverty and of child-specific material deprivation. The international community should be mobilized regarding these ideals and international institutions should consider healthcare to be a global priority like other social rights and contribute to a sustainable development of all countries through peaceful means (The Fund for Peace 2018).

Conclusion

The universal right of access to healthcare of appropriate quality is a civilization-based right from both individual and social viewpoints. A healthy society is a more cohesive, more balanced, and a more productive one. In recent decades, cultural and economic globalization has resulted in a sustained increase in well-being on a global scale. Similar international efforts to implement human rights in a more accelerated manner should also exist. If the rights of cultural minorities are currently in the global political agenda, then social rights such as healthcare access should also be a priority, notwithstanding the fact that they are welfare rights that demand citizens' solidarity. Humanity will be more equal in the future only with the universalization of social rights (Vasak 1977).

Although the global poverty rate declined considerably between 1990 (37.1) and 2015 (9.6) (The World Bank 2016), the contribution of the international community will still be an important step to overcome global disparities between rich and poor countries and to solve many problems related to lack of food, education, shelter, and health in the latter. Moreover, because this improvement is only partial, it is frequently conveyed by nongovernmental organizations and not by states (Global Impact 2016). Both an increase in those contributions and the countries' specificities should be considered so that the international financing of social goods is efficient and effective. Thus, specific cases of international policy should be directed to the needs of each country. Indeed, if food, education, shelter, and health are considered as basic human rights, then they are universal, inalienable, interdependent, and should be internationally guaranteed (Office of the United Nations High Commissioner for Human Rights 2006).

I believe that the existence of a universal right to healthcare access of appropriate quality should not be only an aspirational right but a concrete one. Indeed, this proposal does not question the sovereignty of nation-states in any way. Rather, each nation-state should specify the entitlements of such a right and resource allocation should be performed considering the opportunity cost of different social choices. If all human rights impose different types of obligations on nation-states, namely the need to take positive steps to its fulfillment, then no change in global governance is needed for this right to be fulfilled.

The proposed EO(F) appears to be an ethical and even politically acceptable solution for the existing variable geometry because it allows for different levels of healthcare provision and promotes an ethical rationing while fully respecting accountability for reasonableness (Daniels 2015). This approach also allows for different levels of priorities in healthcare that are context dependent. For instance, it is possible to prioritize healthcare in Norway or in South Africa with the EO(F) as an ethical background. Indeed, and for various reasons, even developed countries need to implement some sort of framework to fairly establish healthcare priorities, despite a significant improvement in socioeconomic development indicators of modern democracies over the past decades. Gender equality in healthcare provision is a good example (European Commission 2019) so that in the future, the implementation of the universal right to healthcare would be gender sensitive.

It is beyond the scope of this chapter to determine how the universal right of access to healthcare of appropriate quality may be propelled in countries and communities that have other social needs beyond healthcare. However, the power of international institutions and of a global ethical conscience may be a good starting point. Indeed, this basic right is a fundamental humanitarian value that should be enjoyed by all citizens of all countries and the members of the international community should recognize the obligation to promote these ideals through any available means.

Note

1   A previous version of this chapter was published in the *Journal of Public Health* in coauthorship with Sofia B. Nunes and Guilhermina Rego.

References

Abel-Smith B. 1994. *An introduction to health: Policy, planning and financing*. Prentice Hall, London.

Brock G. 2009. *Global justice: A cosmopolitan account*. Oxford University Press, Oxford.

Choices in Healthcare. 1992. *A report by the government committee on choices in healthcare*. Choices in Healthcare, The Netherlands.

Council of Europe. 1996. *Convention for the protection of human rights and dignity of the human being with regard to the application of biology and medicine: Convention on human rights and biomedicine*. Council of Europe, Strasbourg.

Daniels N. 1985. *Just healthcare. Studies in philosophy and health policy*. Cambridge University Press, New York.

Daniels N. 1998. Is there a right to healthcare and, if so, what does it encompass? A companion to bioethics. *Blackwell companions to philosophy*, H Kuhse and P Singer (Editors). Blackwell Publishers, Oxford.

Daniels N. 2008. *Just health: Meeting health needs fairly*. Cambridge University Press, New York.

Daniels N. 2015. A progressively realizable right to health and global governance. *Health Care Analysis* 23: 330–340.

Daniels N, Light D and Caplan R. 1996. *Benchmarks of fairness for healthcare reform*. Oxford University Press, New York.

Daniels N and Sabin J. 1997. Limits to healthcare: Fair procedures, democratic deliberation, and the legitimacy problem of insurers. *Philosophy & Public Affairs* 26 (4): 303–350.

Daniels N and Sabin J. 1998. The ethics of accountability in managed care reform. *Health Affairs* 17 (5): 50–65.

Daniels N and Sabin J. 2002. *Setting limits fairly*. Oxford University Press, New York.

Daniels N, Teagarden J and Sabin J. 2003. An ethical template for pharmacy benefits. *Health Affairs* 22 (1): 125–137.

Deloitte. 2011. *The next phase: Opportunities in China's pharmaceuticals market*. Deloitte Touche Tohmatsu CPA Ltd., Shanghai.

European Commission. 2019. Gender equality strategy. Achievements and key areas for action. https://ec.europa.eu/info/policies/justice-and-fundamental-rights/gender-equality/gender-equality-strategy_en [Accessed 12 January 2021].

Ferraz O. 2020. *Health as a human right: The politics and judicialization of health in Brasil*. Cambridge University Press, Cambridge.

Friedman A. 2008. Beyond accountability for reasonableness. *Bioethics* 22 (2): 101–112.

The Fund for Peace. 2018. *2018 Fragile states index*, JJ Messner (Editor). The Fund for Peace, Washington, DC.

Gallego G, Taylor SJ and Brien JA. 2011. Setting priorities for high-cost medications in public hospitals in Australia: Should the public be involved? *Australian Health Review* 35 (2): 191–196.

Gibson J, Martin D and Singer P. 2002. Priority setting for new technologies in medicine: A transdisciplinary study. *BMC Health Services Research* 2: 14.

Global Impact. 2016. http://charity.org/workplace-giving/charity-partners.

Gostin L and Meier B (Editors). 2020. *Foundations of global health and human rights*. Oxford University Press, New York.

Hasman A and Holm S. 2005. Accountability for reasonableness: Opening the black box of process. *Health Care Analysis* 13 (4): 261–273.

Held D. 1995. *Democracy and the global order: From the modern state to cosmopolitan governance*. Polity Press, Oxford.

Human Development Report 2020. 2020. *The next frontier. Human development and the Anthropocene*. United Nations Development Programme, New York.

Ireland-Piper D and Wolff L. 2017. *Global governance and regulation. Order and disorder in the 21st century*. Routledge, London.

Jansson S. 2007. Implementing accountability for reasonableness. The case of pharmaceutical reimbursement in Sweden. *Health Economics, Policy and Law* 2 (2): 153–171.

Kapiriri L, Norheim OF and Martin DK. 2007. Priority setting at the micro-, meso- and macrolevels in Canada, Norway and Uganda. *Health Policy* 82 (1): 78–94.

Kelleher P. 2014. Beneficence, justice and healthcare. *Kennedy Institute of Ethics Journal* 24 (1): 27–49.

The Lancet. 2012. The struggle for universal health coverage. *The Lancet* 380: 859.

Leathard A. 2000. *Healthcare provision. Past, present and into the 21st century*. Stanley Thornes, Cheltenham, 2nd edition.

Meier B and Gostin L. 2018. *Human rights in global health: Rights-based governance for a globalizing world*. Oxford University Press, New York.

Mullen P and Spurgeon P. 2000. *Priority setting and the public*. Radcliffe Medical Press, Abingdon.

Nunes R, Nunes SB and Rego G. 2017. Healthcare as a universal right. *Journal of Public Health* 25: 1–9.

Nunes R and Rego G. 2014. Priority setting in healthcare: A complementary approach. *Health Care Analysis* 22: 292–303.

Nussbaum M. 2009. Creating capabilities: The human development approach and its implementation. *Hyparia* 24 (3): 211–215.

Office of the United Nations High Commissioner for Human Rights. 2006. *Frequently asked questions on a human rights-based approach to development cooperation*. United Nations, New York and Geneva. (H/PB/06/08) www.ohchr.org.

Persad G and Emanuel E. 2017. The case for resource sensitivity. Why it is ethical to provide cheaper, less effective treatments in global health. *The Hastings Center Report* 47 (5): 17–24.

Pogge T. 2008. *World poverty and human rights*. Polity Press, Cambridge, 2nd edition.

Rawls J. 1971. *A theory of justice*. Harvard University Press, New York.

Rego G, Brandão C, Melo H and Nunes R. 2002. Distributive justice and the introduction of generic medicines. *Health Care Analysis* 10: 221–229.

Rid A. 2009. Justice and procedure: How does "accountability for reasonableness" result in fair limit-setting decisions? *Journal of Medical Ethics* 35: 12–16.

Rotberg R. 2003. Failed states in a world of terror. *Foreign Affairs* 81 (4): 127–140.

Sackett D. 2000. *Evidence-based medicine: How to practice and teach EBM*. Churchill Livingstone, London, 2nd edition.

Sahu S. 2014. Globalization, WTO, and the Indian pharmaceutical industry. *Asian Affairs: An American Review* 41: 172–202.

Sen A. 1989. Development as capabilities expansion. *The Journal of Development Planning* 19: 41–58.

Sen A. 1999. *Development as freedom*. Knopf, New York.

Sen A. 2009. *The idea of justice*. Harvard University Press, Cambridge.

Shue H. 1980. *Basic rights: Subsistence, affluence and U.S. foreign policy*. Princeton University Press, Princeton.

Syrett K. 2008. NICE and judicial review: Enforcing "accountability for reasonableness" through the courts? *Medical Law Review* 16 (1): 127–140.

Teagarden J, Daniels N and Sabin J. 2003. A proposed ethical framework for prescription drug benefit allocation policy. *Journal of the American Pharmaceutical Association* 43 (1): 69–74.

Tobin J. 2012. *The right to health in international law*. Oxford University Press, Oxford.

Treaty of Lisbon amending the Treaty on European Union and the Treaty establishing the European Community, signed at Lisbon, 13 December 2007. *Official Journal of the European Union*, C 306, 17 December 2007.

Vasak K. 1977. A 30 year struggle. The sustained efforts to give force of law to the Universal Declaration of Human Rights. *UNESCO Courier*, November, pp. 29–32. https://unesdoc.unesco.org/ark:/48223/pf0000048063 [Accessed 15 January 2021].

Veeder NW and Peebles-Wilkins W. 2001. *Managed care services. Policy, programs and research*. Oxford University Press, New York.

Venkatapuram S. 2009. *Health justice: An argument from the capabilities approach*. Wiley-Blackwell, London.

Venkatapuram S. 2011. *Health justice*. Polity Press, Cambridge.

Wall A and Owen B. 1999. *Health policy*. Gildredge Social Policy, The Gildredge Press, Eastbourne.

Williams I, Robinson S and Dickinson H. 2012. *Rationing in healthcare. The theory and practice of priority setting*. The Policy Press, University of Bristol, Bristol.

Wiseman V, Mooney G, Berry G and Tang K. 2003. Involving the general public in priority setting: Experiences from Australia. *Social Science and Medicine* 56: 1001–1012.

Wolff J. 2012. *The human right to health*. W.W. Norton and Co, New York.

The World Bank. 2016. Development goals in an era of demographic change, global monitoring report 2015/2016, Washington, DC. DOI: 10.1596/978-1-4648-0669-8.

4 Priorities in Healthcare[1]

Most developed countries try to associate economic growth with the provision of certain social services, thus aiming at progressively improving the well-being of citizens. Accordingly, social welfare models have been developed to guarantee that everyone has access to healthcare and education, among other things. In most modern countries, public healthcare keeps improving regarding both treatment outcomes and the patient point of view (Health Consumer Powerhouse 2018). However, there has been progressive growth in public expenditure in the healthcare sector for various reasons, particularly the aging of the population. In 2018, approximately 80% of the healthcare expenditure in modern countries was supported by the taxpayers (OECD 2018). This fact inevitably implies that limits must be established for the public provision of healthcare. Further, in most developed countries, that is, in the Organization for Economic Co-operation and Development (OECD) countries, the proportion of total government expenditure for healthcare is growing steadily.

With the establishment of priorities in healthcare, a more effective adjustment is possible between the demand for and supply of healthcare (National Quality Forum 2014). Explicit forms of rationing have already been implemented in some countries to improve the management of the considerably high public health expenditure, as is the case in Scandinavian countries, the Netherlands, England, and Canada, among others (Choices in Health Care 1992). Some of these prioritization systems resort to a proposal by Norman Daniels known as accountability for reasonableness (Daniels and Sabin 2002), which is an indispensable tool in approaching this matter.

Nevertheless, even if this method provides the required legitimacy to make decisions regarding options in healthcare, the degree of fairness involved in these choices has been questioned. In fact, Daniels bases their proposal on two presuppositions. First, the WHO's health concept is too vast to achieve the appropriate choices in healthcare. Second, and following from the first one, is that fairness in healthcare basically implies attaining a *normal* level of human performance and that the citizens' preferences that do not correspond to the real health requirements need not be met. This chapter aims to try to adjust the accountability for reasonableness to the WHO's holistic view of health and propose an evolutionary method in relation to the *normal* functioning standard proposed by Daniels. This

DOI: 10.4324/9781003241065-5

method contributes to an even more just and equitable prioritization system in healthcare (Nunes and Rego 2014).

Choices in Healthcare: From Legitimacy to Fairness

There are several solutions to overcome the lack of sustainability in public health-care systems, although rationalization and efficiency measures should not be neglected and continue to be implemented. Considering the presupposition that the possibility of increasing the contributions in the form of co-payments is very limited (due to high tax burden in many countries), the combination between efficiency and prioritization in healthcare has enabled the principle of equality regarding the access to healthcare by everyone to be maintained in developed countries. Therefore, in later years, the establishment of priorities in healthcare has been considered in many modern countries regarding the reform of public healthcare systems. The citizens' increasing needs associated with aging and the consequent demographic inversion have led to discrepancies between the demand and supply in healthcare (Williams et al. 2012).

Accountability for reasonableness is probably the most widespread model of priority setting in healthcare in the developed world. In the United Kingdom, for instance, accountability for reasonableness helped shape thinking about how the NICE (National Institute for Health and Care Excellence (2003)) should incor-porate social value judgments into its evidence-based clinical proposals (Syrett 2008). Indeed, public health systems with public accountability, such as those of Canada, the United Kingdom, New Zealand, and Sweden, are now explicitly applying this framework of accountability for reasonableness (Hasman and Holm 2005; Friedman 2008; Kapiriri et al. 2007; Mattei 2016). In the universal coverage systems of most developed countries, such decisions are made by public agencies. In mixed systems, such as in the United States, decisions about whether to fund new developments in drugs, devices, or procedures are made by both public agen-cies and private insurers and managed care organizations. Different solutions have been suggested to overcome the difficulty of many politicians to make controver-sial rationing decisions (Rosén et al. 2014). At a micro level, for instance in the emergency department, the Manchester Triage is universally considered as a fair and appropriate method of selecting patients with different expected prognosis and therefore of explicitly establishing priorities (Manchester Triage Group 1997).

The problem of formal legitimacy (both democratic and public) is usually guaranteed by accountability for reasonableness, but there remains a problem of substantive legitimacy and whether justice as fairness is really considered (Rid 2009). For instance, in the context of NICE and other regulators that have direct impacts on limit setting in healthcare, it has been overtly suggested that a more inclusive process might lead to a solution to the problem of substantive legitimacy. A decision-making process based on inclusive deliberation as an accepted stand-ard of decision-making by the overall democratic society might add fairness to the system (Wall and Owen 1999). It follows that rational decision-making cannot be achieved on the near-exclusive basis of quantitative evidence, and regulators should abide to communitarian values, including most ethical, moral, and religious traditions.

Assuming that countries in a pluralistic society are at least partially neutral, in the sense that every perspective of human happiness has the same relative weight, most regulators adopt a procedural approach to ethics rather than a substantive one (Leathard 2000). Justice is more related to fair procedures and public accountability than to any specific view of the distribution of benefits and burdens. Indeed, a better framework for prioritizing healthcare could be achieved through the inclusion of ethical traditions that give more weight to features that are specific to particular people, communities, families, and political units. In a modern pluralistic society, it is desirable to channel the different views of a good life through rational democratic deliberation through democratic institutions and to directly empower the people.

Qualitative evidence will only partially allow for procedural justice in the deliberative process of healthcare regulators. This process in a democratic society should be objective, comparable, accountable, and externally evaluated. Evidence-based medicine (EBM) is consistent with these principles at a global level, which makes it so appealing and a determinant factor in accountability for reasonableness. As stated by Daniels and Sabin (2002), public accountability means a robust disclosure of relevant information about benefits and performance as well as a demand for due process. A specific array of conditions should be met to comply with the principle of accountability (Daniels and Sabin 2002):

(a) Publicity condition: decisions regarding both direct and indirect limits to care and their rationales must be publicly accessible,

(b) Relevance condition: The rationales for limit-setting decisions should aim to provide a reasonable explanation of how the organization seeks to provide value for money in meeting the varied health needs for a defined population under reasonable resource constraints. Specifically, a rationale will be reasonable if it appeals to evidence, reasons, and principles that are accepted as relevant by fair-minded people who are disposed to finding mutually justifiable terms of cooperation,

(c) Revision and appeals condition: There must be mechanisms for challenge and dispute resolution regarding limit-setting decisions, and, more broadly, opportunities for revision and improvement of policies in the light of new evidence or arguments,

(d) Regulative condition: There is either voluntary or public regulation of the process to ensure that previous conditions are met.

As genetic fingerprints, this framework has both the deliberative process necessary to establish the legitimacy of the decision-making process and the fairness of such decisions (Nunes et al. 2011). Daniels claims that accountability for reasonableness makes limit-setting decisions in healthcare not only legitimate but also fair. But what is really meant by fairness in limit-setting decisions? Daniels argues that claims to equality of opportunity may be limited by scarcity of resources, but nevertheless, choices and priorities in healthcare must be accountable to demo-cratic procedures.

This perspective of distributive justice and its democratic accountability is responsible for the scope and limits of healthcare services. Particular entitlements to healthcare, namely expensive innovative treatments and medicines, may be fairly restricted as long as this decision is socially accountable and imposed by financial restrictions of the system (Nunes 2003). This framework has been used, for instance, in rationing pharmaceuticals in an accountable way (Teagarden et al. 2003) as the process facilitates a broader public discussion about fair limit setting (Daniels et al. 2003).

The starting point of Daniel's account of fairness (Daniels 1985) is that "disease and disability restricting the range of opportunities that would otherwise be open to individuals" are properly seen as unjust and not only as unfortunate circum-stances. As this argument goes the right to healthcare access and delivery does exist as a determinant to the exercise of the equal opportunity rule. This claim for equal opportunity of all citizens intends to ensure *normal* and not a truly *equal* functioning. This distinction seems to be paramount because each one person is not equal to a fellow citizen in the strict sense; in fact, we are entitled to some primary goods that would allow us to function physically, psychologically, and socially at a basic level. Then, our talents and capacities, following our will, may or may not be expressed, depending on the particular circumstances. Further, soci-ety has a moral duty to provide for the necessary means so that anyone is allowed to develop their full potential and expand all their capacities (Sen 1999, 2009). Therefore, as a positive welfare right, the right to healthcare access of appropriate quality imposes on society the duty to allocate resources to health-related needs with maximal efficiency.

This perspective is based on a health concept that is distinct from the WHO's proposals since 1946. Concerning this aspect, Norman Daniels indi-cates, "since we believe that health is a distinct concept from happiness, we also reject the overly broad view of health as a 'state of complete physical, mental, and social well-being,' and not merely the absence of disease or infir-mity," which is embodied in the WHO's definition (Daniels et al. 1996). By *normal* performance, we mean the performance of the average citizen (a cri-terion for the reasonable person). Excellent or truly equal performance is not the case since such a radical view of the citizens' equal rights contradicts the proper essence of human diversity. That is, "We correct for some 'natural' effects on that distribution – disease and disability – but we do not attempt to eliminate all differences in the name of a radically expansive view of equal opportunity" (Daniels et al. 1996).

The question then is how distributive decision-making in healthcare may gain in fairness by giving wider representation to the diversity of perspectives in con-temporary societies. Specifically, the meaning of *normal* functioning or behavior itself is a matter of controversy. This is the reason why the WHO's definition of health is such a broad concept. Meanwhile, there is no hierarchy in the provi-sion of health when the standard is *normal* versus *non-normal* functioning. Even in *normal* functioning criteria, some treatments and medical interventions have priority over others. For instance, prioritizing heart attack over a mild pain in the knee can be hardly disputed, although both conditions deserve accurate diagnosis and treatment.

Justice might be advanced with a progressive approach because in principle, every health service (treatment, diagnosis, and so on) might be negotiated in the deliberative process (Gold 2009). But fairness is also optimized because the confluence between vertical and horizontal equity implies that, even within the basic package, a progressive approach leads to a true hierarchy of priorities, meaning that a particular treatment has precedence over another, even though the latter may still be an integral part of the basic package. This is a valuable tool both in the hospital setting and in primary care (O'Neill et al. 2018). This rationale should also be applied in the interface between healthcare delivery and public health protection. For instance, in low- and middle-income countries, although important health gains have been obtained, relatively low coverage of highly cost-effective health interventions (such as universal vaccination) has been delivered, spending the scarce resources on high-cost, less effective care (Glassman and Chalkidou 2012).

Equal Opportunity Function: A Complementary Approach?

To enable better compatibility between accountability for reasonableness and the integrated view of health of the WHO, a change of paradigm is suggested regarding the referential *all or nothing* such as proposed by Daniels (*normal* versus *non-normal* functioning) (Daniels 1998). Although the logical consequence of justice as fairness is the implementation of an effective opportunity for everyone to have access to healthcare of appropriate quality, it should imply the existence of a universal and general healthcare system. However, its revaluation in light of a distributive justice may dictate a different future (Figure 4.1).

Equal opportunity may be represented graphically in the form of the equal opportunity function, (EO)F. This involves the convergence between the concepts of vertical and horizontal equity. The philosophical and economic scope of these concepts does not specify the relevant properties to characterize an agent as equal. If it is necessary to treat equals in the same manner regarding the distribution of material resources and others in an unequal manner, it is essential to define a method that enables this distinction to be established. The graphic representation of (EO)F in the theoretical plan uses two variables:

1   The X-axis represents the variable hierarchy of needs in accordance with the Maslow pyramid (physiological, safety, belongingness and love, esteem, self-actualization, and self-transcendence needs).
2   The Y-axis indicates the healthcare performance level, which reaches a maximum value through the universality of access and comprehensiveness of public services and a minimum value when the access to healthcare services is the individual responsibility of each citizen.

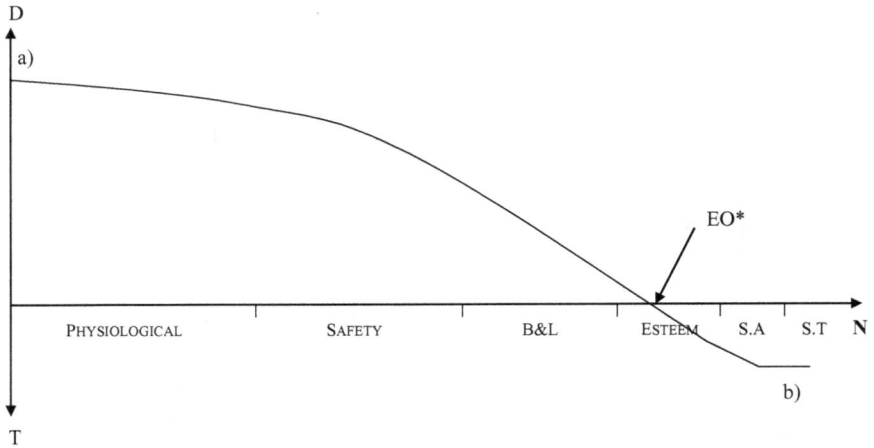

D

a)

EO*

PHYSIOLOGICAL   SAFETY   B&L   ESTEEM   S.A   S.T   N

b)

T

LEGEND:

D: Healthcare Delivery
T: Tiering
N: Needs (Maslow)
B&L: Belongingness and Love
S.A: Self-Actualization
S.T: Self-Transcendence

Figure 4.1 Equal Opportunity Function (EO)F – WHO Version.

When (EO)F intersects the X-axis (point EO*), in accordance with the combination of the needs criteria and the financial restrictions imposed by the system, there appears a point from which the provision of healthcare through public services is not strictly mandatory. From this point, any citizen may have access to healthcare at the cost of their own individual responsibility or the professional group to which they belong without damaging the principle of justice as fairness if they resort to alternative coverage schemes, namely private health insurance or out-of-pocket payments. But this is the case only if the fulfillment of the second-order needs may be at issue, which may be situated schematically and in a variable form, as from the point that Maslow defined as esteem needs (in comparison with the *normal* functioning criteria; see Figure 4.2).

Daniels establishes a distinction between health *need* and health *preference*, which is a distinction between the healthcare needs to reach a level of physical and psychological functioning typical of our species, and mere preferences or conveniences that are beyond a reasonable and consensual level of normality. Although it is not possible to satisfy all esteem and self-actualization needs, nor all individual preferences, it is up to each person to use their financial resources (individual responsibility) to achieve this objective. From point EO*, and even in an ideal society with absolute availability of resources in which these needs can be

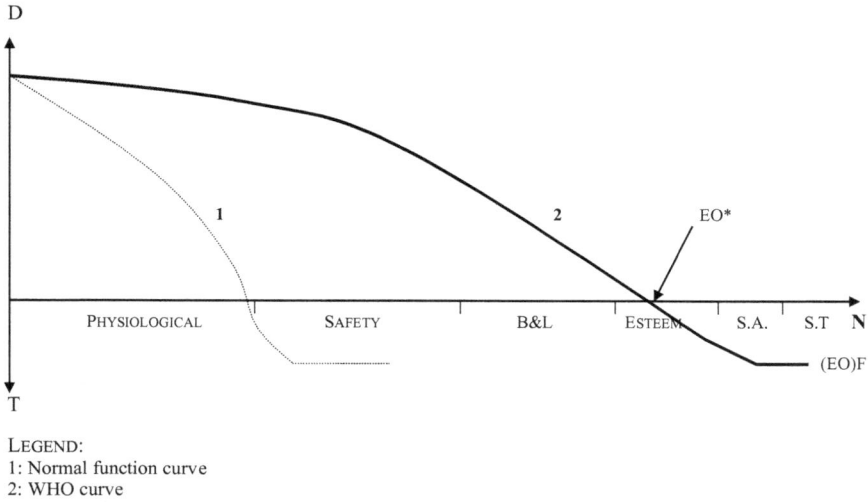

LEGEND:
1: Normal function curve
2: WHO curve

Figure 4.2 Equal Opportunity Function (EO)F – "Normal Function" Version.

met, it is not only an option but even likely a duty to proceed with prioritization in the present state of economic and financial restriction. In practice and presupposing a maximum efficiency of the public healthcare systems, (EO)F allows for the establishment of priorities in healthcare as far as the health services at issue aim at meeting the needs that do not interfere with the normal performance of a citizen.

The universality of access is not subject to any objection, but the claim that there are no limits to public provision (with individual needs being almost unlimited as major criteria by definition) is currently contested since the allocation of society's resources to health must compete with the supply of other social goods (social cost of opportunity). Indeed, one of the major challenges of modern societies is to converge economic development with human development, and therefore, it has been overtly suggested that a true developed society promotes every aspect of human fulfillment, such as health, education, and gender equality (Human Development Report 2018). Inevitably, a delicate balance emerges between the social goods that the citizens may or may not be entitled to in conformity with the social and economic situation of a particular society. According to Penelope Mullen and Peter Spurgeon (2000), "The demand for healthcare is infinite, and so rationing is inevitable." Thus, prioritizing has become the conceptual paradigm of the health policies of developed countries (Mullen and Spurgeon 2000).

Inequality (treating two people in a different way) becomes inequity (treating two people in an unfair way) if a solid motive does not exist to justify the negative discrimination of a citizen to the detriment of another. However, the opposite is equally valid; that is, an apparent inequity becomes a mere inequality (ethically acceptable and, therefore, fair) if it conforms with the restrictions imposed on the system with the application of economic constraints that are consistent with the (EO)F. But this is only the case if and only if that situation of inequality does not harm citizens' basic rights and if the process that led to the decision is democratically determined while conforming with public accountability criteria.

Reformulating this perspective of the problem, the restrictions of an economic and financial nature transform a decision for allocation of resources from iniquitous (unfair) to acceptable (fair) as far as it does not negatively discriminate any class of citizens, even though a particular class of services may be legitimately restricted. This seems to be a huge dilemma for health systems: to articulate the right of access to the necessary and appropriate healthcare in a fair and impartial manner using the resources available in society. To illustrate this proposal, we refer to the application of the (EO)F to elective cesarean delivery.

EBM has focused on particular aspects of medicine, and specific areas (such as elective on-demand cesarean delivery) have been left behind because there is some difficulty in performing this kind of EBM research (Nama and Wilcock 2011). Although there is still no absolute evidence about the risk/benefit analysis of on-demand cesarean delivery, EBM must be carefully evaluated in this setting if adequate health policies are to be promoted (Nygaard and Cruikshank 2003). Evidence should be obtained by international cooperation and by independent agencies so that the goals are truly achieved (National Institutes of Health 2006; WHO 2018). This evidence is necessary for fair resource allocation policy to be accomplished. Indeed, even if it is accepted that there is a right to reproductive autonomy, allowing a woman to make informed choices about pregnancy and birth, another issue is related to the social costs of this kind of decision (Boerma et al. 2018). Therefore, it should be clearly determined whether it should be included in the basic healthcare package or if it should be left to individual responsibility.

From an ethical perspective, on-demand cesarean delivery faces a problem of justice in the allocation of healthcare resources. In a changing economic environment, it is not surprising that new approaches to healthcare may limit the provision of care as it is not possible to deliver everything to everyone. As there is no absolute evidence about the comparative risks and benefits of vaginal versus abdominal deliveries (Sandall et al. 2018; Keag et al. 2018), because many studies focus on side effects of cesarean section performed due to clinical reasons and not on-demand, we will focus specifically on the relevance condition as far as the rationale, reasons, and principles for limit-setting decisions are concerned. Indeed, choices and priorities in healthcare are fair if they are accountable to democratic procedures. Daniels states quite clearly:

> In any healthcare system, then, some choices will have to be made by a fair, publicly accountable, decision-making process. Just what constitutes a fair decision-making procedure for resolving moral disputes about healthcare entitlements is itself a matter of controversy. It is a problem that has been addressed little in the literature. Our rights are not violated, however, if the choices that are made through fair decision-making procedures turn out to be

ones that do not happen to meet our personal needs, but instead meet needs of others that are judged more important.

(Daniels 1998)

This perspective of distributive justice and its democratic accountability is responsible for the scope and limits of healthcare services. Particular entitlements to healthcare, namely access to a particular type of delivery in a public service, may be fairly restricted as long as the decision is socially accountable and subject to financial restrictions of the system. In many countries, for instance, upper- and middle-class women regularly choose abdominal deliveries during childbirth since they can afford to pay for it in private clinics. In the private healthcare system, where women come from higher levels of income and education, cesarean delivery prevails. In contrast, in the public sector, where women belong to less privileged social classes, vaginal deliveries are the usual practice due to medical care routines that are imposed on them.

In principle, a pregnant woman's reproductive autonomy should be respected. For instance, the 2011 NICE guideline states, "For women requesting a CS [cesarean section], if after discussion and offer of support . . . a vaginal birth is still not an acceptable option, offer a planned CS" (National Institute for Health and Clinical Excellence 2011). Nevertheless, as far as the rationale and the reasons for limit setting are concerned, Daniels' relevance condition implies that thorough economic analysis should be performed. Imposing a restriction to the basic package in healthcare necessarily implies that the competitive medical treatment (on-demand cesarean delivery) is more expensive than the usual one (vaginal delivery). If the price is the same or lower, then there is no reason based on fairness to restrict its use in public services (although it may be restricted by a risk/benefit analysis).

This economic analysis should consider not only direct costs but also indirect ones. In cesarean versus vaginal delivery, only the unitary price of each procedure, as determined by each country's health authority (or insurance company), is usually considered. In general, the unitary price mainly reflects the aggregated costs of the professionals, the operating room, and the materials used. However, this analysis may be biased because the cost of a cesarean delivery is usually calculated for cesareans performed with medical indications (crash cesareans for instance), which tend to be much more expensive than cesarean on-demand, which are planned and elective.

Indeed, most reports show that the cost of cesarean delivery is higher than vaginal birth. Therefore, one may claim that the practical application of the (EO) F can place cesarean delivery in the T segment (tiering) of the Y-axis; that is, outside the basic healthcare package. Then, public healthcare systems have the responsibility to promote good-quality planned parenthood services. However, some interventions, such as on-demand cesarean delivery, may be legitimately beyond the scope of the basic package (Lindstöm and Waldau 2008). Pregnancy and birth are consistent with Daniels' *normal* functioning and thus, are health needs, not a mere preference. Nevertheless, the proposed methodology, the (EO) F, allows for a fairer decision-making process in this circumstance. Meanwhile, in the future, if it is economically demonstrated that the cost of vaginal birth is higher than that of a cesarean delivery, a straightforward application of the (EO)F may show that cesarean section may be included in the basic package. The (EO) F curve will then have great elasticity regarding the number of services available to all citizens, allowing for fair adjustment of the basic package to the resources allocated to healthcare.

Conclusion

Undoubtedly, health systems must be explicit about prioritization. Norman Daniels' theory of justice in healthcare is the most widespread tool to accomplish this goal. However, it faces a practical problem in how to allocate resources fairly when they are especially scarce. Daniels claims that accountability for reasonableness makes limit-setting decisions in healthcare not only legitimate but also fair.

This chapter has assessed the latter claim. Does accountability for reasonableness result in fair limit-setting decisions? Different options have been discussed for resolving this lack of clarity. Further, the ways they apply to Daniels' accountability for reasonableness framework is also examined. In general, this theory holds that treatments that accomplish a *normal* species-typical behavior should be in the basic package and that this is accepted by reasonable people. Therefore, a treatment that does not relate to a health need, but only to an individual preference, should be left out (Gallego et al. 2011).

The presented proposal offers an evolution from this perspective. For instance, preimplantation genetic diagnosis (PGD) is not strictly essential for a person's normal functioning. Nevertheless, if there are enough resources available, this method of diagnosis can be still offered to the general public. Access to PGD will contingently depend on the balance reached by the social contract between the global number of resources and the public services desired. Then, the (EO)F curve is not static but slides to the left or right depending on particular social arrangements. That is, in principle, with growing resources, more health services can be included in the basic package (moving the (EO)F curve to the right), while during scarcity, the amount of health services can be reduced (moving the (EO)F curve to the left).

What about prioritizing treatments that are considered in normal function but are more expensive than other alternatives (such as on-demand cesarean section, some medical-assisted procreation technologies, some blood alternatives, or snoring surgery in non-pathological cases)? Moreover, does the traditional framework of accountability for reasonableness help to prioritize pharmaceuticals that have proven medical benefits but are extremely expensive in a just and fair way (Jansson 2007; Gibson et al. 2002)? How far should society be involved in these decisions so that they are legitimate and fair (Wiseman et al. 2003)?

It can be claimed that applying the WHO's definition of health in setting priorities can allow access to a wider range of healthcare without violating the four conditions underlying accountability for reasonableness. Indeed, publicity, revision and appeals, and regulative conditions are mainly procedural conditions but are extremely useful in legitimizing healthcare choices by applying the (EO)F. The relevance condition may even be optimized with this rationale because one can claim that not only a *reasonable* explanation but also a *fair* explanation should be given for how value for money is optimized.

In the European tradition, the (EO)F appeals to evidence, reasons, and principles that may be accepted as fair by most citizens. The Manchester Triage System (MTS) is a practical example of the (EO)F at a micro level. From a justice perspective, the MTS algorithm implies that more fundamental needs (such as protecting life) have priority over less fundamental ones, although the latter may also be considered. At a macro level, the (EO)F can be not only fairer but also more practical because it will also allow for a more equitable management of waiting lists if the reasons and the rationale for choices are made public and are truly accountable.

Thus, accountability for reasonableness is an extremely valuable tool to address the issue of setting limits in healthcare. Further, the (EO)F can reflect how accountability for reasonableness results in fair limit-setting decisions. However, this methodology must be further specified to best achieve such decisions. Indeed, when resources are especially scarce (as in low-income countries), the methodology suggested in this chapter can not only allow prioritizing on an all-or-nothing basis but also contribute to a more systematic and fairer approach. It may even be considered as an evolutionary perspective in relation to Daniels' account of fairness.

In developed societies, most citizens are aware of the need to establish priorities in healthcare. However, there is strong disagreement about the ethical legitimacy of many choices. That is why different frameworks of ethical decision-making have been suggested, such as rationing through inconvenience (Eyal et al. 2018) or through collaboration and shared values (Sabin 2018). The *normal* functioning standard suggested by Daniels is very appealing because a reasonable and prudent person can easily determine what services should be included in the basic package. However, this standard may leave important modalities of diagnosis and treatment out of public services. The (EO)F evolves from this perspective: a gradual approach and a true hierarchical system of priorities in healthcare can be enabled by considering a distinction regarding the treatments that may or not be included in the basic package.

Moreover, as suggested in Chapter 3, this approach is of variable geometry in the sense that the (EO)F may adapt to any society and to very different levels of development. Indeed, this model is easily responsive to the economic and budgetary specificities of a given population if basic healthcare is guaranteed to every citizen. However, it is not unfair that low- and middle-income countries have a basic healthcare package that is not as comprehensive as the package of more developed societies. If the decision-making process is fair and accountable, it should be supported by global governance institutions such as the WHO.

Note

1 A previous version of this chapter was published in *Health Care Analysis* in co-authorship with Guilhermina Rego.

References

Boerma T, Ronsmans C, Melesse DY et al. 2018. Global epidemiology of use of and disparities in caesarean sections. *The Lancet* 392: 1341–1348.

Choices in Health Care. 1992. *A report by the government committee on choices in health care.* Choices in Health Care, The Netherlands.

Daniels N. 1985. *Just health care. Studies in philosophy and health policy.* Cambridge University Press, New York.

Daniels N. 1998. Is there a right to health care and, if so, what does it encompass? A companion to bioethics. *Blackwell companions to philosophy*, H Kuhse and P Singer (Editors). Blackwell Publishers, Oxford.

Daniels N, Light D and Caplan R. 1996. *Benchmarks of fairness for health care reform.* Oxford University Press, New York.

Daniels N and Sabin J. 2002. *Setting limits fairly.* Oxford University Press, New York.

Daniels N, Teagarden J and Sabin J. 2003. An ethical template for pharmacy benefits. *Health Affairs* 22 (1): 125–137.

Eyal N, Romain P and Robertson C. 2018. Can rationing through inconvenience be ethical? *The Hastings Center Report* 48 (1): 10–22.

Friedman A. 2008. Beyond accountability for reasonableness. *Bioethics* 22 (2): 101–112.

Gallego G, Taylor SJ, Brien JA. 2011. Setting priorities for high-cost medications in public hospitals in Australia: Should the public be involved? *Australian Health Review* 35 (2): 191–196.

Gibson J, Martin D and Singer P. 2002. Priority setting for new technologies in medicine: A transdisciplinary study. *BMC Health Services Research* 2: 14.

Glassman A and Chalkidou K. 2012. *Priority-setting in health. Building institutions for smarter public spending. A report of the center for global development's priority-setting.* Institutions for Global Health Working Group, Washington, DC.

Gold M. 2009. Engaging the American people in setting healthcare priorities. *Patients, the public and priorities in healthcare*, P. Littlejohns and M. Rawlins (Editors). Radcliffe Publishing, Oxford.

Hasman A and Holm S. 2005. Accountability for reasonableness: Opening the black box of process. *Health Care Analysis* 13 (4): 261–273.

Health Consumer Powerhouse. 2018. *Euro health consumer index 2017 report.* Health Consumer Powerhouse, Stockholm.

Human Development Report. 2018. *Human development indices and indicators.* 2018 Statistical Update. http://hdr.undp.org/en/2018-update/download.

Jansson S. 2007. Implementing accountability for reasonableness. The case of pharmaceutical reimbursement in Sweden. *Health Economics, Policy and Law* 2 (2): 153–171.

Kapiriri L, Norheim OF and Martin DK. 2007. Priority setting at the micro-, meso- and macrolevels in Canada, Norway and Uganda. *Health Policy* 82 (1): 78–94.

Keag OE, Norman JE and Stock SJ. 2018. Long-term risks and benefits associated with cesarean delivery for mother, baby, and subsequent pregnancies: Systematic review and meta-analysis. *PLoS Medicine* 15: e1002494.

Leathard A. 2000. *Health care provision. Past, present and into the 21st century.* Stanley Thornes, Cheltenham, 2nd edition.

Lindstöm H and Waldau S. 2008. Ethically acceptable prioritisation of childless couples and treatment rationing: "Accountability for reasonableness". *European Journal of Obstetrics & Gynecology and Reproductive Biology* 139 (2): 176–186.

Manchester Triage Group. 1997. *Emergency triage.* BMJ Publishing, London.

Mattei P. 2016. *Public accountability and health care governance. Public management reforms between austerity and democracy.* Palgrave Macmillan, Basingstoke.

Mullen P and Spurgeon P. 2000. *Priority setting and the public.* Radcliffe Medical Press, Abingdon.

Nama V and Wilcock F. 2011. Caesarean section on maternal request: Is justification necessary? *The Obstetrician and Gynaecologist* 13 (4): 263–269.

National Institutes of Health. 2006. NIH state-of-the-science conference statement on caesarean delivery on maternal request. *NIH Consens State Sci Statements* 23: 1–29.

National Institute for Health and Care Excellence. 2003. *A guide to NICE.* National Institute for Health and Care Excellence, London.

National Institute for Health and Care Excellence. 2011. *Caesarean section, Issued: November 2011, NICE clinical guideline 132.* National Institute for Health and Care Excellence, London. guidance.nice.org.uk/cg132.

National Quality Forum. 2014. *Priority setting for healthcare performance measurement: Addressing performance measure gaps in care coordination.* Final Report August 15, 2014. National Quality Forum, Washington DC.

Nunes R. 2003. Evidence-based medicine: A new tool for resource allocation? *Medicine, Health Care and Philosophy* 6 (3): 297–301.

Nunes R, Brandão C and Rego G. 2011. Public accountability and sunshine healthcare regulation. *Health Care Analysis* 19 (4): 352–364.

Nunes R and Rego G. 2014. Priority setting in health care: A complementary approach. *Health Care Analysis* 22: 292–303.

Nygaard I and Cruikshank DP. 2003. Should all women be offered elective cesarean delivery? *Obstetric Gynecology* 102 (2): 217–219.

OECD. 2018. *Spending on health.* Latest trends. www.oecd.org/els/health-systems/Health-Spending-Latest-Trends-Brief.pdf. Organization for Economic Co-operation and Development, Paris.

O'Neill B, Aversa V, Rouleau K, Lazare K, Sullivan and Persaud N. 2018. Identifying top 10 primary care research priorities from international stakeholders using a modified Delphi method. *PLoS One* 13 (10): 1–10. https://doi.org/10.1371/journal.pone.0206096.

Rid A. 2009. Justice and procedure: How does "accountability for reasonableness" result in fair limit-setting decisions? *Journal of Medical Ethics* 35: 12–16.

Rosén P, Licht J and Ohlsson H. 2014. Priority setting in Swedish health care: Are the politicians ready? *Scandinavian Journal of Public Health* 42 (3): 227–234. https://doi.org/10.1177/1403494813520355.

Sabin J. 2018. Rationing care through collaboration and shared values. *The Hastings Center Report* 48 (1): 22–36.

Sandall J, Tribe RM, Avery L et al. 2018. Short-term and long-term effects of caesarean section on the health of women and children. *The Lancet* 392: 1349–1357.

Sen A. 1999. *Development as freedom.* Knopf, New York.

Sen A. 2009. *The idea of justice.* Harvard University Press, Cambridge.

Syrett K. 2008. NICE and judicial review: Enforcing "accountability for reasonableness" through the courts? *Medical Law Review* 16 (1): 127–140.

Teagarden J, Daniels N and Sabin J. 2003. A proposed ethical framework for prescription drug benefit allocation policy. *Journal of the American Pharmaceutical Association* 43 (1): 69–74.

Wall A and Owen B. 1999. *Health policy*. Gildredge Social Policy, The Gildredge Press, Eastbourne.

Williams I, Robinson S and Dickinson H. 2012. *Rationing in health care. The theory and practice of priority setting*. The Policy Press, University of Bristol, Bristol.

Wiseman V, Mooney G, Berry G and Tang K. 2003. Involving the general public in priority setting: Experiences from Australia. *Social Science & Medicine* 56: 1001–1012.

World Health Organization. 2018. *WHO recommendations non-clinical interventions to reduce unnecessary caesarean sections*. World Health Organization, Geneva.

5 Evidence-Based Medicine and Resource Allocation

Evidence-based medicine (EBM) is defined as the conscious and judicious use of current best evidence in making decisions about the care of individual patients. A greater level of evidence implies a higher recommendation grade. This pioneering explicit concept of EBM as a helpful tool for both patients and physicians is embedded in a particular view of medical practice: the singular nature of the patient–physician relationship and the commitment of the physician toward their client's health. This view (often labeled as Hippocratic after the name of the Greek physician) rests upon a unique tradition in medical practice. There is no doubt that it is a value-laden definition that focuses on an individual's quality of care. Moreover, it is well known that physicians hold to their beliefs very strongly, claiming that it is unethical not to do so. Physicians need clear and objective information based on randomized clinical trials and meta-analytic studies, but diagnosis and treatment will remain subjective because of the psychological dimensions of the patient–physician relationship (Nunes 2003).

Nevertheless, in many modern countries this "integration of the best evidence from systematic research with clinical expertise and patient values" (Sackett et al. 2000) appears to be reinterpreted in view of the scarcity of healthcare resources. In fact, from a public policy perspective, the EBM is increasingly regarded as intrinsically prescriptive. In this vein, some authorities claim that EBM is a new paradigm for medical practice (Howick 2011) and that medicine as an art and healing profession is outdated as opposed to the objectiveness of treatment evaluated via randomized clinical trials.

One of the main reasons that EBM is so necessary is the existence of large amounts of dispersed human research, but with no global diffusion. Further, the avenues through which science is delivered are frequently questioned due to a lack of ethical safeguards. Indeed, medicine should be centered on research that is clinically relevant, that is, both basic and clinical research. Studies of particular interest include diagnosis, treatment, and prognosis. EBM usually relies upon a definition of the clinical question to be researched, selection of evidence, critical methodological evaluation of the evidence, synthesis, and application. Indeed, the scientific method produces data that are the basis of scientific evidence. This approach is the best-known way to diminish random or systematic biases and must be used for clinical decision-making.

DOI: 10.4324/9781003241065-6

The purpose of this chapter is twofold: first, to show that EBM should guide clinical practice from an ethical perspective in accordance with the principles of beneficence and scientific integrity. Second, to show that EBM may be a useful tool in the macro-allocation of healthcare resources.

Research, Integrity, and Choices in Healthcare

Biomedical research involving human subjects is a common practice worldwide. However, this practice still provokes anxiety among the public. Indeed, since the late 1960s, individual physicians have been unable to cope with some ethical dilemmas in research involving human subjects due to severe breaches of scientific integrity. Moreover, the large amount of published science makes people question the validity of the findings, especially when they report very different results. For example, more than 50 million medical articles are available in different databases.

Stringent guidelines have been proposed to regulate different types of human research. According to the Council for International Organizations of Medical Sciences (CIOMS 2002), the following types of research must be regulated:

1   Studies of physiological, biochemical, or pathological processes or responses to specific interventions (physical, chemical, or psychological) in healthy subjects or patients;
2   Controlled trials of a diagnostic, preventive, or therapeutic measure in larger groups of persons designed to demonstrate a specific generalizable response to these measures against the background of individual biological variation;
3   Studies designed to determine the consequences of specific preventive or therapeutic measures for individuals and communities; and
4   Studies concerning human health-related behavior in a variety of circumstances and environments.

It is also frequently argued that specific legislation should exist to protect vulnerable human subjects in accordance with accepted guidelines and recommendations. These principles are mainly procedural, notwithstanding the fact that different ethical backgrounds are involved in its foundation (National Commission for the Protection of Human Subjects of Biomedical and Behavioral Research 1978). They can be summarized as follows:

1   Respect for persons and the need for free and informed consent,
2   Protection of vulnerable persons, including children and psychiatric patients (surrogate decision-making, proxy consent, living will, etc.),
3   The ethical imperative to maximize benefits and minimize harm (beneficence and non-maleficence),
4   Privacy rights, confidentiality, and the right to be forgotten,
5   Justice and equity in access to healthcare and the benefits of clinical trials (Bankowski et al. 1997),

6   Accountability of healthcare professionals and institutions delivering health-
     care (Nunes et al. 2009), and
7   Responsibilities of ethical review committees.

Another binding principle is respect for personal autonomy and informed consent
(Nunes 2016). The ethical and legal doctrine of informed expressed consent is
a means to respect the individual patient and to enforce the ethical principles
of autonomy and beneficence. Written consent (documented consent) is usually
required, and ethics committees are empowered to control this consent over time
(written consent is a legal requirement in most countries). In epidemiological
studies, both the individual and the entire community were evaluated. Obtaining consent is advisable; however, this is sometimes impossible. The International
Ethical Guidelines for Epidemiological Studies (CIOMS 2002) clearly states that
the ethical review committee should determine whether it is ethically acceptable to proceed without individual informed consent in epidemiological research.
Securing the agreement of the authority responsible for public health in a specific
population is a necessary but not sufficient condition. Ethics committees play a
major role in epidemiological research because they guarantee that this research
will be conducted following general ethical standards.

Specific legislation should exist to protect both competent and vulnerable subjects in accordance with accepted guidelines and recommendations, namely the
Convention for the Protection of Human Rights and Dignity of the Human Being
with Regard to the Application of Biology and Medicine (Council of Europe 1996).
The international harmonization of legislation is necessary. Issues such as stem
cell and embryo research, eugenic abortion, human gene therapy, human genetic
enhancement, synthetic biology, health databases, and biobanks (World Medical Association 2016) also need careful consideration from international regulatory bodies so that ethics committees are aware of legitimate patterns of behavior.
Clinical trials should abide by these principles in a transparent and accountable
manner (Nunes et al. 2011).

There is also a clear distinction between clinicals trials across phases I, II, III,
and IV. As a rule, phase IV clinical trials are considered the normal evaluation of
a new pharmaceutical product that has been recently approved by the governmental agency. In phase IV, clinical trials are usually not submitted to an extensive ethical review process. However, there are no differences between phase I,
II, and III clinical trials because they are all considered potentially hazardous to
human subjects. Similar stringent guidelines have been applied. Scientific review
committees should exist in all hospitals and research facilities to help deal with
these issues. Ethics committees must frequently deal with dilemmas within specific groups of subjects. A controversial issue with no clear answer is the ethics of
research in vulnerable patients.

Research on children is questioned because valid consent is impossible, and
children are particularly vulnerable. However, if medicine is to progress, pediatric
research must be performed. If parental consent is obtained (the long-standing
principle of familial autonomy), then most pediatricians feel that research can and

should be performed. However, more stringent guidelines are required. One of these guidelines refers to the distinction between therapeutic and nontherapeutic clinical trials. Usually, the law considers nontherapeutic clinical trials in children unethical, and therefore, unlawful under any circumstances. An accepted guideline refers to a social understanding of the best interests of a child. Any child has at least the right to their autonomy, and society should provide the means to fulfill the right to an open future. The existence of this right was first proposed by Joel Feinberg (1980), referring to the concept of *rights-in-trust*, that is, rights that are to be saved for the child until they are an adult. These rights must be protected in the present to be exercised later in life. This general category of rights holds that parents do not own their children but are rather only guardians on their behalf.

A child's scope of future choices must be protected (Nunes 2001). Article 29th of the World Medical Association (2013) Declaration of Helsinki states clearly that:

> When a potential research subject who is deemed incapable of giving informed consent is able to give assent to decisions about participation in research, the physician must seek that assent in addition to the consent of the legally authorized representative. The potential subject's dissent should be respected.

The use of both children and adults as controls in randomized controlled trials is a common and accepted practice worldwide. These controls are critical for consistent scientific conclusions. At least two unresolved ethical dilemmas are likely to be addressed soon by ethical review committees: autonomy and the right to choose between being randomized or not, and the ethical adequacy of using control subjects at all (*versus* using information previously gathered from historical controls). Statutory regulations should address these issues.

Regarding clinical trials, legislation usually requires that the review process and recommendations be compulsory; researchers must follow the committees' suggestions to meet ethically accepted standards. However, in the clinical setting, the committee usually makes recommendations in accordance with national and international laws and regulations. Nevertheless, clinicians still have a wide range of decision-making capacity. This optional basis is the core of the case review practice. Indeed, medical ethics implies that professionals are independent in their judgment and any intrusion in the clinical practice may severely affect the patient–physician relationship. The challenge is even greater because many members of ethics committees are not physicians themselves. This *recommendation model* is the best possible practice to accommodate ethical advice with the best clinical outcome (even at physician request), especially when subjectivity is a well-known factor underlying the patient–physician relationship. In addition, experimental treatments that have not been screened using a stringent EBM methodology, such as innovative cancer treatment modalities, may require urgent approval by the ethics committee. In the future, if the amount of work of ethics committees becomes unbearable, then professional ethics committees can be considered.

Ethics committees face new challenges in future clinical trials. Fundamental human rights to dignity, personal liberty, and identity could be violated more subtly. If this is the case, then more stringent guidelines are needed to protect the human subject. Importantly, most ethics committees deal with clinical trials; therefore, the complex methodology of scientific analysis must also be evaluated. Questions such as the role of statistics and the goals of epidemiological investigation must be answered. The rights of vulnerable patients should also be preserved. The rights of future generations, especially regarding the right to inherit a genetic endowment that has not been artificially disrupted, should also be addressed (Melo et al. 2001).

Despite these ethical guidelines, a lack of integrity is a major problem that helps motivate EBM. Values such as personal integrity are paramount. Integrity is a fundamental aspect of human life; it is an intimate sphere that cannot be manipulated or coercively undermined. It is the proper foundation of the human person and is rooted in convictions about what is most valuable in life. Issues such as the professional standards of conduct must be addressed. Indeed, there is a lack of integrity when a scientist's specific behavior questions the validity of the research (Peels and Bouter 2018). Misconduct and questionable research practices may have different motivations. Some conflicts of interest are usually at stake, namely, when a secondary interest takes over the primary interest. According to the Australian Medical Association,

> A conflict of interest occurs when a particular relationship or practice gives rise to two or more contradictory interests; that is, when the various interests that guide their decisions or behaviors can potentially generate conflicting outcomes. . . . The specific case of a conflict of interest in medicine that is of particular concern is that which arises when a doctor has professional or personal interests, whether pecuniary or non-pecuniary, or relationships that may lead them to make professional judgments that are in conflict with their primary responsibility to their patient.
>
> (AMA 2018)

Secondary interests may be related to material gains, intellectual and scientific credit, or even personal credit. For instance, the European Code of Conduct for Research Integrity suggests different settings in which integrity should be promoted (ALLEA 2017):

1   Research environment,
2   Training, supervision, and mentoring,
3   Research procedures,
4   Data practices and management,
5   Collaborative working,
6   Publication and dissemination,
7   Reviewing, and
8   Evaluating and editing.

Honesty in all aspects of research and appropriate accountability arrangements in the conduct of research are paramount (World Conference on Research Integrity 2010). In addition, responsible research and innovation relies on EBM for proper development in every aspect of research, including epidemiologic studies. Swaen et al. (2018) suggest that

> epidemiologic research has had and is likely to continue to have an important role in evidence-based public health and clinical medicine. Epidemiological research findings have greatly contributed to improving human health by identifying risk factors, evaluating preventive programs, determining the best treatments for disease and care, and providing insight into prognostic factors. Given the limited resources available, it is of great importance that biomedical research is conducted according to the best feasible scientific standards. Epidemiology studies cannot be done without the participation of patients or healthy volunteers who invest their time and participate in studies they believe are performed according to the highest feasible standards.

Codes of conduct are an important tool to explain and identify the right behavior. However, the scientific system should adapt itself in accordance with the principles and guidelines of EBM so that fabrication, falsification, and plagiarism are downgraded to residual levels. Responsible conduct of research implies that every piece of scientific research should be reproducible and that valid negative studies should also be published. Indeed, original studies cannot be trusted if they cannot be reproduced. The promotion of preprint and post print peer reviews should also be a common practice in science. The validity and reliability of science should prevail over the secondary interests of researchers. It follows that a curriculum in ethics and responsible research is needed at the pre-graduate level in all healthcare professions. The fiduciary bond between society and the research system should be changed to always consider citizens' well-being and the health of the patient as the first consideration of physicians and other researchers.

Evidence-Based Medicine and Societal Goals

EBM may have different societal and healthcare goals depending on the overall understanding of the common good and the role of the state as a redistributor of resources (vertically and horizontally). The individual physician assumes an important and responsible place in systems where access to healthcare services is mainly left to individual responsibility (through out-of-pocket payments or managed care/insurance mechanisms) and where solidarity is not felt as a social obligation (Horne 2017). However, again, the patient–physician relationship is a common endeavor between these two agents (or more if it is an incompetent patient) as this relationship is grounded in the ethical principles of beneficence and non-maleficence. Thus, respect for personal autonomy is a part of the clinical process and is usually considered to be a necessary but not sufficient condition for the accomplishment of the intended clinical outcome. State intrusion in this

intimate sphere is troublesome and is admitted only to the extent of macro decisions of social and political relevance. In this model, EBM can be a tool to help
clinicians decide on the best available evidence and avoid litigation by strictly
adhering to specific guidelines. The justified and responsible departure from these
guidelines is thus not considered unethical (or unlawful) because the bio-psycho-
social construct of disease and illness captures the individual nature of this process. Moreover, managed care integrates EBM as an important management tool
that distills healthcare services to be provided on a contractual basis.

However, in many countries, the welfare state emerging from World War II led
to the assumption that health (and its protection) is not only an individual right
but also a social good because an investment in public health leads to social cohesion. Therefore, it is claimed that there is a basic right of access to healthcare of
appropriate quality (Nunes et al. 2017). In most modern countries, for instance,
this social contract is visible through social medicine measures, leading to the
existence of a National Health Service (NHS) or some other kind of universal
health coverage (Palfrey 2000). This order helps ensure this right. Participating
countries have a primary duty to:

1   Guarantee the access of all citizens, regardless of their economic circum-
    stances, to both preventive and curative care;
2   Guarantee a rational and efficient coverage of healthcare resources through
    the whole country;
3   Provide the costs of medical care and medicines from public funds within
    limits set by democratic procedures; and
4   Regulate and supervise privately funded medical practice by coordinating it
    with the public system to ensure that adequate standards of efficiency and
    quality are achieved in public and private institutions.

Solidarity is a social principle that enables governments to coerce tax citizens and
accomplish social goods. Intergenerational solidarity through the taxation of a specific segment of the population guarantees the financing of most social goods. As
stated in the Report by the Government Committee on Choices in Health Care,
Ministry of Welfare, Health, and Cultural Affairs of the Netherlands (Choices in
Health Care 1992),

> solidarity is the awareness of unity and a willingness to bear the consequences
> of it. Unity indicates the presence of a group of people with a common history
> and common convictions and ideals. Solidarity can be voluntary, as when
> people behave out of humanistic motives, or compulsory as when the govern-
> ment taxes the population to provide services to all.

Solidarity has a different historical background. It can be found, although with different names, in Catholic and Protestant traditions as well as in Marxist, socialist,
and even libertarian thinking. It is deeply grounded as the most modern healthcare
system, both as a doctrine and as a political choice. This perspective, grounded in

egalitarian and utilitarian values, is usually regarded as instrumental in achieving equality of opportunity and access to primary social goods.

In this context, the confluence of public health values with EBM will likely lead to its compulsory use. The pressure of this change may lead to EBM's usage not only in the clinical setting but also as a resource-allocation instrument. EBM may even be an imperative for the responsible physician, even if clinical autonomy is diminished. In fact, the patient–physician relationship is essentially a trust-based enterprise; freedom regarding the choice of different therapeutic options is the usual practice. EBM must be integrated with the patient's individual circumstances (psychological, familial, and social), leading to the best possible clinical outcomes. The medical profession must be aware that the usual standard of good medical practice is *leges artis*, a concept determined by evidence-based data more than ever. Indeed, according to Gibson et al. (2005),

> Evidence-based medicine (EBM) focuses on effectiveness and appropriateness in allocating resources for health services to particular patient populations. When resources are scarce, clinical evidence can help to make allocation decisions that minimize waste of resources on ineffective or inappropriate treatments and maximize use of resources on the right treatment for the right patient at the right time.

From a public health perspective, EBM should try to reconcile opposing views of distributive justice and its translation to clinical practice, that is, the classical/ Hippocratic paradigm of medicine along with the social model in which the clinician is just one among other actors in healthcare delivery (Smith 1994). Note that evidence-based public health is not synonymous with EBM as a public health tool. The latter means that EBM is a useful instrument in public policy (Yip and Hafez 2015). The former translates the EBM methodology, namely, the search for evidence, to public health interventions. This implies that the search for evidence is also paramount in this domain. A fair healthcare system will embrace both EBM and evidence-based public health as tools to promote efficiency and effectiveness.

Ultimately, EBM implementation must constructively engage stakeholders around a new healthcare policy. If EBM succeeds, healthcare professionals, other providers, healthcare organizations, and society at large must be carefully explained of the expected benefits for the individual patient clinical care and the rationale behind its implementation.

Evidence-Based Public Policy

It is frequently claimed that healthcare needs are infinite, and therefore, efficient allocation of resources and prioritization are inevitable in public healthcare systems. If we accept the principle of equity in healthcare access, meaning that the material principle of justice involved in the distribution of wealth is mainly based on personal needs (Powers and Faden 2000), a reduction of unjust disparities between individual citizens or social groups is paramount. As a political option, equity has different social and economic implications: equity insofar as resources are allocated, in the way healthcare services are received, and in the way those services are paid for (CIOMS 1997). Different foundations do exist regarding claims of equity. All these try to fulfill the formal principle of justice that equals must be treated equally, in the exact measure of its similarity or dissimilarity. There are several competing theories of justice that are regarded as the proper foundation of equity and fair equality of opportunity in healthcare access and delivery.

The libertarian Robert Nozick claims that property rights and liberty are paramount in a fair society. Fair procedures (procedural justice in acquisition, transfer, and rectification) should guarantee these rights; state intrusion is only accepted to protect them. The redistribution of private property through taxation is regarded as unjust (usually viewed as equivalent to forced labor). Healthcare is not considered a right under this theory (Nozick 1974). In contrast, John Rawls' difference principle (Rawls 1971, 2001) argues that both liberty and fair equality of opportunity (equity) must be considered. Nevertheless, some social and economic inequalities are permitted if the greatest benefit of the least advantaged is pursued. In the healthcare context, this egalitarian theory of justice implies the existence of a decent minimum of healthcare; however, tiering is allowed, in principle, if access to the lower level is not undermined. Notably, utilitarian views of justice are the basis of most welfare systems of healthcare delivery. If society is better off with a fair distribution of resources, then utility is maximized; this is probably because such an approach promotes social cohesion and provides security to its citizens. Thus, the distribution of basic healthcare to all citizens is usually accepted on utilitarian grounds. Regardless of the interpretation of the principle of equity, most healthcare systems accept different, even contradictory, material principles of justice in practice. In fact, principles specifying relevant properties for distribution, such as need, effort, contribution, or merit of the subject, or those claiming an equal share or a free-market exchange, are usually put into practice in most developed countries' social systems.

Resource allocation plays an important role in healthcare delivery, notwithstanding the fact that medical practice has developed steadily in the last decades in both scientific knowledge and technological levels. Long-standing principles, such as the physician as an autonomous agent, physicians treat patients who are sick or ill, not diseases, or the patient–physician relationship as an enterprise based on trust, should be reinterpreted considering the role of the state as a redistributor of resources at least insofar as healthcare access is concerned. It must be clearly explained to the medical profession that the first objective of EBM is not to limit the scope of medical intervention but rather to increase scientific knowledge and therefore, to increase the quality of care.

The second objective is to allocate resources as fairly as possible and to uphold the treatments of unproven clinical results. In this way, both the individual and community will benefit. This course of action is a consequence of the acceptance of health as a social good and the overall responsibility of healthcare agents toward society. Access to healthcare is limited by the scarcity of resources. Treatments with unproven efficacy and effectiveness should not be included in the basic package. This package is financed by the solidarity of taxpayers and must truly contribute to the global improvement of health at both the individual and social levels. Citizens have the right to know how policy-makers spend their taxes on healthcare.

Although health is a major individual right, it must compete for resources with other social goods, including education, job training, and environmental protection. Thus, resources should be spent as efficiently as possible because any allocation decision (opportunity cost) clearly affects other important social rights. EBM may be instrumental insofar as macro-allocation decisions are concerned. Economical assessment and effectiveness evaluation of new technologies are now the usual practice in many developed countries. The British National Institute for Health and Care Excellence (NICE) is a good example of this new public policy. Nevertheless, choices and priorities in healthcare must be accounted for by democratic procedures (Staley 2001). Norman Daniels (1998) states quite clearly that

> In any healthcare system, then, some choices will have to be made by a fair, publicly accountable, decision-making process. What constitutes a fair decision-making procedure for resolving moral disputes about healthcare entitlements is itself a matter of controversy. This problem has been addressed only slightly in the literature. Our rights are not violated, however, if the choices that are made through fair decision-making procedures turn out to be ones that do not happen to meet our personal needs, but instead meet the needs of others that are judged more important.

This perspective of distributive justice and democratic accountability is responsible for the scope and limits of healthcare services. Particular entitlements to healthcare, that is, expensive innovative treatments and medicines, may be fairly restricted as long as this decision is socially accountable and imposed by the financial restrictions of the system. A fortiori, the implementation of EBM is in accordance with this perspective if it limits access to drugs and treatments of unproven scientific results (Honigsbaum et al. 1997). The primary goal of most countries with EBM in terms of drug policy is for universal access based primarily not only on personal needs but also on contribution; thus, access is indirectly reflected in merit and effort or even free-market transactions.

Access to pharmaceuticals as well as the overall healthcare policy is grounded in an accepted right to healthcare access, notwithstanding the fact that priorities must be set even in the access to useful medicines. Further, in a global environment of health research, health biotechnology will challenge the ethical limits of any healthcare system at the national and global levels (Zhenzhen et al. 2004). Indeed, any healthcare system will face the pressure of emerging technologies, which must be carefully evaluated both in publicly financed systems and in more liberal ones (Kaebnick and Gusmano 2018). Precision medicine is a good example of this.

Nevertheless, in the global environment of resource allocation, EBM's usage to restrict apparently useful clinical treatments, on the grounds of both a lack of scientific evidence and a distributive justice requirement, can be a useful tool to facilitate the access of all citizens to a reasonable level of healthcare and to promote the system's efficiency (Taylor 1998). Moreover, from a medical ethics perspective, it may be in accordance with the long-standing tradition of beneficence in clinical practice. In fact, there is a clear distinction between *resource allocation* and *a saving money policy*. EBM implementation may even increase healthcare expenditure, but scarce resources will be then allocated more fairly to treatments of proven benefit (Figure 5.1).

Even individual physicians, including both general practitioners and specialists, rely much more on EBM than on opinion-based medicine. This paves the way for a new approach in clinical practice. This approach is fundamental to increasing the health status of most patients. However, EBM has not focused on specific areas that may be left behind because there is simply no interest or possibility to perform EBM research, such as long-term care. Thus, EBM must be carefully evaluated in clinical practice because the pharmaceutical industry is more prone to investigate areas that are more economically profitable (Gascón et al. 2017). EBM should also be performed via international cooperation and via independent agencies (such as Cochrane) to achieve its goals. Otherwise, EBM may even increase healthcare expenditure because evidence may probably only exist for new and expensive treatments.

The existence of evidence per se might be an important factor driving new healthcare needs. From a health economics perspective, new needs will lead to a

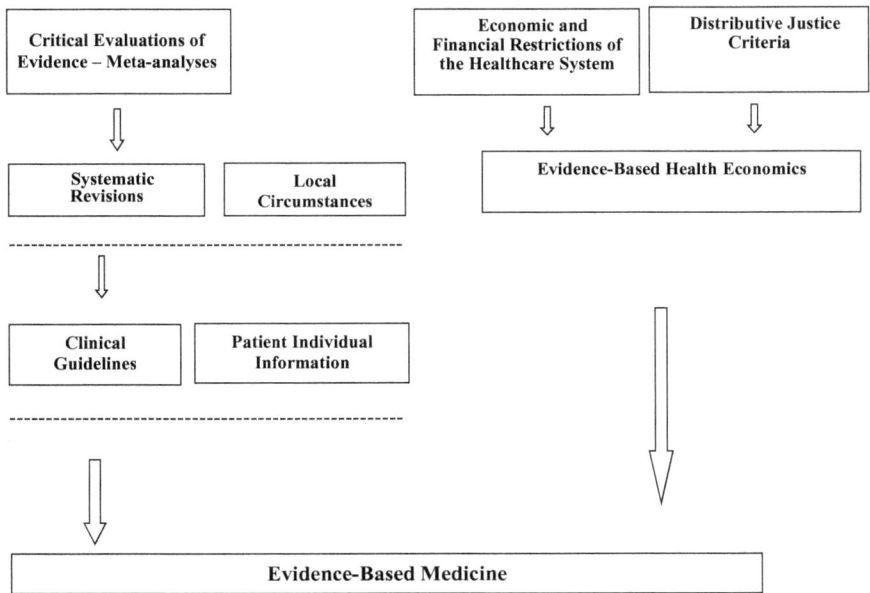

Figure 5.1 Evidence-Based Medicine and Resource Allocation.

greater demand for healthcare services. Another determining factor in the adoption of EBM in clinical practice is pressure from managed care through private insurance companies (Veeder and Peebles-Wilkins 2001). It has been common practice to uphold any treatment, medical or surgical, if it does not comply with international EBM-grounded standards. This policy has at least two different motives: resource allocation and litigation avoidance. These and other forms of managed care must be in accordance with the accepted principle of public accountability so that people can know for sure what kind of services are delivered and who should control these services (Nunes and Rego 2014).

Conclusion

Most healthcare professionals welcome EBM, especially general practitioners. It may even increase its credibility within society. However, there are lingering questions about what to do if a specific EBM guideline does not meet patients' expectations (and there is no available effective option). It is also unclear how to proceed if the patient is worse-off with a treatment modality suggested by a particular guideline. Professional and managed care liability should be addressed by experts in this field. If EBM is used as a resource-allocation tool, it should embrace not only drug policy but also new areas of research such as individualized treatment via pharmacogenetics. It will be necessary to demonstrate the efficacy and effectiveness of the intervention; biased and fragmented information in this domain will challenge the imagination of EBM specialists because of the individual nature of pharmacogenetics (as in many other areas of health biotechnology), like other areas of personalized and precision healthcare.

In parallel with its clinical endeavor, EBM also plays a fundamental role as a resource-allocation instrument. Nevertheless, both clinicians and clinical epidemiologists try to adopt a neutral position regarding resource-allocation policies. However, there is no doubt that, as suggested by Penelope Mullen and Peter Spurgeon (2000), "if the rationing of scarce resources requires resources to be targeted at the most effective interventions, it is necessary to have appropriate evidence as to which these are." Further, as stated by Daniels et al. (1996), "the healthcare we have strongest claim to is care that effectively promotes normal functioning by reducing the impact of disease and disability thus protecting the range of opportunities that would otherwise be opened to us."

In conclusion, while EBM is a useful tool for clinicians, it is critical to develop health policies that address the overall problem of scarcity in healthcare resources. The criteria for prioritizing healthcare, namely the widespread principle of accountability for reasonableness (Daniels and Sabin 1998), will demand that services and treatments be included in the public service. These are, more than ever, evidence based. Clinical practice as well as research and teaching should embrace this new paradigm to its full extent to accomplish these goals (Straus et al. 2018).

References

ALLEA. 2017. *The European code of conduct for research integrity*. All European Academies (ALLEA), Berlin. www.allea.org/publications/joint-publications/european-code-conduct-research-integrity/.

AMA. 2018. AMA guidelines for doctors on managing conflicts of interest in medicine 2018. *Australian Medical Association*. https://ama.com.au/position-statement/guidelines-doctors-managing-conflicts-interest-medicine-2018.

Bankowski Z, Bryant J and Gallagher J. 1997. *Ethics, equity and health for all*. Council for International Organizations of Medical Sciences, (CIOMS) Geneva.

Choices in Health Care. 1992. A report by the government committee on choices in health care. Choices in Health Care, The Netherlands.

CIOMS – Council for International Organizations of Medical Sciences. 1997. *Ethics, equity and health for all*, Z Bańkowski, J Bryant and J Gallagher (Editors). Council for International Organizations of Medical Sciences, Geneva.

CIOMS – Council for International Organizations of Medical Sciences. 2002. *International ethical guidelines for biomedical research involving human subjects*. World Health Organization (WHO), CIOMS, Geneva.

Council of Europe. 1996. *Convention for the protection of human rights and dignity of the human being with regard to the application of biology and medicine*. Council of Europe, Strasbourg. November.

Daniels N. 1998. Is there a right to health care and, if so, what does it encompass? A companion to bioethics. *Blackwell companions to philosophy*, H Kuhse and P Singer (Editors). Blackwell Publishers, Oxford.

Daniels N, Light D and Caplan R. 1996. *Benchmarks of fairness for health care reform*. Oxford University Press, New York.

Daniels N and Sabin J. 1998. The ethics of accountability in managed care reform. *Health Affairs* 17 (5): 50–65.

Feinberg J. 1980. *The child's right to an open future. Whose child? Children's rights, parental authority and state power*, W Aiken and H LaFollette (Editors). Littlefield, Adams & Co., Totowa, NJ.

Gascón F, Lozano J, Ponte B and De la Fuente D. 2017. Measuring the efficiency of large pharmaceutical companies: An industry analysis. *European Journal of Health Economics* 18: 587–608.

Gibson JL, Martin K and Singer PA. 2005. Evidence, economics and ethics: Resource allocation in health services organizations. *Healthcare Quarterly* 8 (2): 50–59.

Honigsbaum F, Holmström S and Calltorp J. 1997. *Making choices for health care*. Radcliffe Medical Press, Oxon.

Horne LC. 2017. What makes health care so special? An argument for health care insurance. *Kennedy Institute of Ethics Journal* 27 (4): 561–587.

Howick JH. 2011. *The philosophy of evidence-based medicine*. Wiley-Blackwell, Hoboken.

Kaebnick G and Gusmano M. 2018. CBA and precaution: Policy-making about emerging technologies. *A Hastings Center Special Report* January–February: 88–96.

Melo H, Brandão C, Rego G and Nunes R. 2001. Ethical and legal issues in xenotransplantation. *Bioethics* 15 (5/6): 427–442.

Mullen P and Spurgeon P. 2000. *Priority setting and the public*. Radcliffe Medical Press, Abingdon.

National Commission for the Protection of Human Subjects of Biomedical and Behavioral Research. 1978. The Belmont Report. Ethical Principles and Guidelines for the Protection of Human Subjects of Research. Government Printing Office, (DHEW publication No. (OS) 78–0012), Washington, DC.

Nozick R. 1974. *Anarchy, state and utopia.* Basic Books, New York.

Nunes R. 2001. Ethical dimension of paediatric cochlear implantation. *Theoretical Medicine and Bioethics* 22: 337–349.

Nunes R. 2003. Evidence-based medicine: A new tool for resource allocation? *Medicine, Health Care and Philosophy* 6 (3): 297–301.

Nunes R. 2016. *Diretivas Antecipadas de Vontade.* Conselho Federal de Medicina, Brasília.

Nunes R, Brandão C and Rego G. 2011. Public accountability and sunshine healthcare regulation. *Health Care Analysis* 19 (4): 352–364.

Nunes R, Nunes SB and Rego G. 2017. Healthcare as a universal right. *Journal of Public Health* 25: 1–9.

Nunes R and Rego G. 2014. Priority setting in health care: A complementary approach. *Health Care Analysis* 22: 292–303.

Nunes R, Rego G and Brandão C. 2009. Healthcare regulation as a tool for public accountability. *Medicine, Health Care and Philosophy* 12: 257–264.

Palfrey C. 2000. *Key concepts in health care policy and planning.* Macmillan Press, London.

Peels R and Bouter L. 2018. The possibility and desirability of replication in the humanities. *Palgrave Communications* 4 (95). www.nature.com/articles/s41599-018-0149-x.

Powers M and Faden R. 2000. Inequalities in health, inequalities in health care: Four generations of discussion of justice and cost-effectiveness analysis. *Kennedy Institute of Ethics Journal* 10 (2): 109–127.

Rawls J. 1971. *A theory of justice.* Harvard University Press, New York.

Rawls J. 2001. *Justice as fairness. A restatement,* E Kelly (Editor). Harvard University Press, Cambridge.

Sackett D, Strauss S, Richardson W et al. 2000. *Evidence based medicine.* Churchill Livingstone, London.

Smith B. 1994. *An introduction to health: Policy, planning and financing.* Prentice Hall, London.

Staley K. 2001. *Voices, values and health. Involving the public in moral decisions.* King's Fund Publishing, London.

Straus S, Glasziou P, Richardson WS and Haynes B. 2018. *Evidence-based medicine: How to practice and teach EBM.* Elsevier, New York, 5th edition.

Swaen G, Langendam M, Weyler J et al. 2018. Responsible epidemiologic research practice: A guideline developed by a working group of the Netherlands epidemiological society. *Journal of Clinical Epidemiology* 100: 111–119. https://doi.org/10.1016/j.jclinepi.2018.02.010.

Taylor D. 1998. *Improving health care. A King's Fund policy paper.* King's Fund Publishing, London.

Veeder N and Peebles-Wilkins W. 2001. *Managed care services. Policy, programs and research.* Oxford University Press, New York.

World Conference on Research Integrity. 2010. The Singapore statement on research integrity. Second World Conference on Research Integrity, Singapore, July 21 to 24, 2010. https://wcrif.org/guidance/singapore-statement.

World Medical Association Declaration of Helsinki. 2013. Ethical principles for medical research involving human subjects, adopted by the 64th WMA General Assembly, Fortaleza, Brazil, October 2013.

World Medical Association Declaration of Taipei. 2016. Ethical considerations regarding health databases and biobanks, adopted by the 67th WMA General Assembly, Taipei, Taiwan, October 2016.

Yip W and Hafez R. 2015. *Improving health system efficiency. Reforms for improving efficiency of health systems: Lessons from 10 countries*. World Health Organization, Geneva.

Zhenzhen L, Jiuchun Z, Ke W et al. 2004. Health biotechnology in China: Reawakening of a giant. *Nature Biotechnology* 22: 13–18.

6   Global Health in a Digital World

Health, when defined as individual well-being, also has a collective dimension since well-being and the absence of disease depend on important community efforts besides individual factors. Hence, the protection of health is an individual obligation as well as a social responsibility of any modern and advanced society. However, today, society is a huge global village (McLuhan and Powers 1989) because economic globalization and consequent cultural harmonization imply a new look at human development.

Thus, health can have a third dimension that is beyond individual and community dimensions to include a global perspective, in the context of transnational organization of efforts and resources, for preventing and controlling diseases whose causes and respective impacts extend beyond politically determined territorial boundaries. Indeed, global health can be also perceived as a tool for global justice (Sen 1999).

Global Health in Perspective

Global health is defined by Koplan et al. (2009) as "the area of study, research and practice that places a priority on improving health and achieving equity in health for all people worldwide." Global health broadly means supranational interdependency for promoting worldwide health in areas where concerted international efforts are effective. This includes tackling infectious diseases that have no borders or other global threats with global economic impact. Therefore, global health can be defined as promotion of health on a global scale and the convergence of efforts to that end. This translates into a gradual improvement in global health indicators, assuming that there is complementarity between national and transnational efforts with a positive impact on the healthcare sector (Engebretsen and Heggen 2015). Measurement and comparisons of disability- and quality-adjusted life years, and mortality rates among different countries are important tools for effective benchmarking on a global scale. For instance, according to the Global Burden of Disease (GBD) 2016 Lifetime Risk of Stroke Collaborators' (2018) study, "the global lifetime risk of stroke from the age of 25 years onward was approximately 25% among both men and women. There was geographic variation in the lifetime risk of stroke, with the highest risks in East Asia, Central Europe, and Eastern Europe."

DOI: 10.4324/9781003241065-7

This view of global health starts with certain ethical assumptions, beginning with health as an essential and a fundamental right that is inherent to human dignity (Nunes et al. 2017). In the absence of effective mechanisms and institutions of global governance, the World Health Organization (WHO) has been the visible face of global health implementation using the best existing evidence, especially regarding the implementation of public health measures and primary healthcare (World Health Organization 2021). The Alma Ata Declaration has been one of the benchmarks of action, mainly in low- and middle-income countries (LMICs). However, according to the WHO, there is a significant shortage of healthcare professionals on a global scale; if this trend continues, this deficit will reach 14 million by 2030.

The United Nations (UN) has also played a decisive role over the past few years through the establishment of the sustainable development goals (SDG) that put health at the epicenter of global policy decisions (United Nations 2021). An accurate analysis shows that health promotion is a specific goal that can also be transversally found in all other goals:

1 End poverty in all its forms everywhere,
2 End hunger, achieve food security and improved nutrition, and promote sustainable agriculture,
3 Ensure healthy lives and promote well-being for all at all ages,
4 Ensure inclusive and equitable quality education and promote lifelong learning opportunities for all,
5 Achieve gender equality, and empower all women and girls,
6 Ensure availability and sustainable management of water and sanitation for all,
7 Ensure access to affordable, reliable, sustainable, and modern energy for all,
8 Promote sustained, inclusive, and sustainable economic growth, full and productive employment, and decent work for all,
9 Build resilient infrastructure, promote inclusive and sustainable industrialization, and foster innovation,
10 Reduce inequality within and among countries,
11 Make cities and human settlements inclusive, safe, resilient, and sustainable,
12 Ensure sustainable consumption and production patterns,
13 Take urgent action to combat climate change and its impacts,
14 Conserve and sustainably use the oceans, seas, and marine resources for sustainable development,
15 Protect, restore, and promote sustainable use of terrestrial ecosystems, sustainably manage forests, combat desertification, halt and reverse land degradation, and halt biodiversity loss,
16 Promote peaceful and inclusive societies for sustainable development, provide access to justice for all and build effective, accountable, and inclusive institutions at all levels, and
17 Strengthen the means of implantation and revitalize the global partnerships for sustainable development.

Other crucial issues include reducing premature mortality rates caused by non-communicable diseases, ensuring universal access to sexual and reproductive health services, ending the epidemics of acquired immune deficiency syndrome (AIDS), tuberculosis, and malaria, and defining strategies to prevent or minimize global pandemics such as SARS-CoV-2. To achieve universal health coverage is another major objective of this program.

Achieving these goals is an ambitious project, given that there is a variable geometry with very different levels of development on the five continents. In fact, the ideal society is one that eliminates all forms of poverty (including hunger), promotes health and well-being, views education as the central pillar of human development, combats all forms of discrimination, and promotes gender equality (Nunes 2020). However, the 21st-century society also values work as an expression of human self-realization and looks at economic and industrial development as a means to achieve happiness and harmony among people. In accordance with the UN, healthcare becomes a public health problem at the national level but also an essential aspect to full human development and the very sustainability of life in the long term. That is, the concept of global health also includes the legitimate rights of future generations along with environmental concerns; for example, climate change will be a decisive factor in global health. Indeed, global health implies a special concern with the commonwealth of life (One Health).

Public health traditionally develops health promotion and prevention strategies in a specific society. This national specificity is understandable as each nation-state has its own territorial, economic, and political organization. Thus, and understandably, initiatives to promote collective health are realized in the context of implementation of other social policies. As we shall see later, each nation-state considers the available resources, implements a specific health system in line with the wishes of the population, and initiates preventive and health promotion measures that are more adequate and responsive to the intended objectives (Nunes and Rego 2014). Health promotion efforts are sometimes made at regional levels, given the costs of implementing modern and effective health policies, and the disparity of possible models and strategies for the implementation of effective public health (GBD 2017 Mortality Collaborators 2018). For example, the European Union (EU) tries to conciliate the different health policies of the 27 member states with a broader view. This allows cross-border mobility of European citizens and helps the EU implement common health promotion policies (European Parliament 2011) and a true European Union for Health. For instance, the European Centre for Disease Prevention and Control (www.ecdc.europa.eu/en) played a major role in combating COVID-19 pandemic.

An example of the need for effective global health is the existence of a national vaccination plan in each country based on WHO recommendations. This plan includes a list of diseases that is constantly updated in accordance with the existing scientific data and the political choices of each society. The list typically includes diphtheria, pertussis, rubella, polio, tetanus, measles, epidemic parotitis, and/or human papilloma, among others. However, in many countries, vaccination is not compulsory as children are not vaccinated against the will of their parents. Nevertheless, the ethical and legal responsibilities of promoting the best interest of the child also rest within this context, and thus, the responsibility to authorize vaccination.

Obviously, this is a very important public health problem since the intention is to achieve universal immunization, bearing in mind that a population is protected only if everyone is immunized (herd immunity). Even in more civilized countries, the existence of some people who have not been immunized can cause major disease outbreaks. Then, one may ask why some parents refuse to vaccinate their children? Some of the most widespread fears about vaccinations include a variety of reasons: a) vaccines cause autism; b) infant immune systems cannot handle so many vaccines; c) natural immunity is better than vaccine-acquired immunity; d) vaccines are not worth the risk; and e) we do not need to vaccinate because infection rates are already so low. An intensive health literacy campaign is therefore essential to inform the population about individual and collective benefits of vaccinations. However, if there is a small group (no matter how small) of unvaccinated people, a Pandora's box will be opened as unvaccinated people easily become contaminated with the disease and transmit it to third parties, thereby preventing universal protection.

Ethically, the doctor should use all possible means to try to persuade parents about the benefits of vaccination for preventing these diseases. Nevertheless, in many societies, parents may refuse to have their child vaccinated. Still, through open and empathetic communication, the doctor should explain the importance of vaccinations and the possible consequences of a person not being vaccinated. There is an appreciable range of diseases that are now extinct or are merely residual in many countries because fortunately, international recommendations for universal vaccination were followed. The focus is to match the best interests of children with existing scientific evidence, thus preventing the occurrence of certain diseases before they manifest themselves. In fact, a universal vaccination program has an enormous impact on public health (Kaslow 2018).

This case well exemplifies the importance of a transnational implementation of a comprehensive vaccination program, under the supervision of WHO, which considers the huge movement of people between different geographical areas. Its benefit is evident to people and society. By preventing the transmission of pathogens, universal vaccination has even eradicated some diseases, such as smallpox. However, vaccinations also have important positive externalities, such as promotion of school attendance or increased corporate productivity.

However, social networks today allow for a high degree of global connectivity, permitting the formation of chains of opinion in a closed circuit with dramatic effects on the decision of many citizens and not only within the so-called extreme communities. Indeed, it is estimated that by 2023, 92% of the global population will have access to the Internet. Therefore, implementation of global health should consider the enormous impact of the digital revolution on all aspects of our lives by facilitating connectivity and posing new challenges, such as protection of individual privacy.

The Rise of Digital Health

The ubiquitous use of online social platforms has generated a profound impact on behavioral health. The concept of vaccinations is just one example among many others (Terrasse et al. 2019). Skin cancer, reproductive health, and pharmaceutical advertising are among other prominent examples. The growth of this *social mediome* even created the need to implement an extensive program of research on the ethical, legal, and social implications of the social media revolution. Even a Hippocratic Oath for tech was proposed. However, according to Kaebnick and Gusmano (2019),

> With record-high cases of measles around the world generating media attention, the Senate holding hearings about the dangers of the anti-vaccination movement, and Facebook (FB) adopting new rules for vaccine-related content, it seems we might be on the verge of squelching vaccine misinformation.

Further, the American Medical Association (2019) recommends special attention when addressing social network systematic use since networking can provide opportunities to widely disseminate beneficial public health messages. Thus, this reinforces the idea that social networks, blogs, and other forms of communication online should be in accordance with specific ethical principles, namely the protection of personal privacy and preservation of the common good (public beneficence).

Besides social networks, the scientific and technological developments over the last decades, namely regarding information and communication technology (ICT), have been transforming the dynamics of the doctor–patient relationship for various reasons. On the one hand, the new information technologies have contributed to cultural globalization and thus, to the overlap of different perceptions of the common good. On the other hand, this democratization in access to information has had a profound impact on the interface between medicine and society. Relevant examples include the use of the Internet as a privileged source of information, the introduction of telemedicine in most health systems in the world, and even the generalization of remote consultations, namely by telephone, email, and Facebook.

Now, there is a consensus that the use of new communication technologies and modern information systems, such as telephone, radio, television, dedicated networks, wireless communication, and biotelemetry (used to monitor the permanence of humans in space by satellite), can bring numerous benefits to the practice of medicine and other healthcare-related professions. The concept of digital health is therefore a very broad one, encompassing the use of ICT, including mobile health (mHealth), health information technology (IT), health information systems, wearable devices, telehealth, telemedicine, machine intelligence, and augmented reality. Telephone consultations, being the most traditional form of ICT use, have some peculiarities that distinguish it from other types of telemedicine, namely the fact that it is a technology in real time and the current practice is not to store information in digital modes or audio recording.

According to the American Telemedicine Association (2019), telemedicine refers to "the use of medical information through electronic communications to improve the health status of patients." Moreover, according to the association, between electronic communications and patients, the concept of telehealth is related with telemedicine but has a broader scope. Telehealth not only refers to clinical services in the strict sense but includes other factors such as e-health. However, the use of IT (email and Internet) that involves collecting, storing, and sending information for analysis (image, signal, and video) has different ethical and legal implications in relation to telephone consultation. This is due to, among other factors, the materialization of results.

The global health community acknowledges the importance of digital technology as a transformational tool for definitively improving global health. According to Taylor and Alper (2018), the three main areas of digital health are as follows:

1   The delivery of health information to health professionals and consumers through the Internet and telecommunications;
2   Using ICTs to improve public health services, such as through education and training of health workers; and
3   Using health information systems to capture, store, manage, or transmit information on patient health or health facility activities.

There is no doubt that digital health can radically transform the health system of any country and has that capacity. This is observable via its high degree of interoperability and by its speed and reach to increase efficiency, effectiveness, and even access to health. However, to be truly effective, it is necessary to integrate and harmonize different digital solutions to gain scale and efficiency. For example, this can be done by integrating different health information systems, such as those of the public and private sectors, and even increasing the connectivity between systems in different countries. Only then will it be possible to better plan new public health strategies and promote better organization of health services worldwide.

However, if the objective is to apply it on a global scale, it is necessary to ensure the system interoperability and to propose appropriate laws to govern digital health. Regulation is deemed essential for the numerous organizations enrolled in planning and development to be effectively supervised. Further, connectivity must respect individual privacy because it is a right that most people want to preserve in modern societies. According to Boman and Kruse (2017),

> Supporting global health goals with information and communications technology (ICT) involves four kinds of access, namely access to the Internet, to individual health data (medical data), to individual data indirectly linked to health, and to data about the environment of the individual, relevant to health.

Further, there are large collections of both structured and unstructured data called big data (and data lake) and questions by society and public authorities over the destiny of this large amount of information and how it can be used to make better decisions for mankind (Kayaalp 2017). Data mining, machine learning (including deep learning and reinforcement learning), machine reasoning (planning, scheduling, knowledge representation and reasoning, search, and optimization), and robotics (integration of different techniques into cyber-physical systems) have been developed to extract information and transform it for a valuable utilization. We must address the importance of big data in global health along with the ethical dilemmas associated with this type of data (Mittelstadt and Floridi 2016). Big data can be characterized by 5 V's (Drosou et al. 2017):

1   Volume,
2   Velocity,
3   Variety,
4   Veracity, and
5   Value.

Big data-associated technologies have the potential to be used in new predictive models in health, risk reduction, and more personalized and precision medicine (Campos et al. 2017). It can also be a fundamental tool in medical research (Ienca et al. 2018). The enormous amount of data existing in different databases, especially if they are interoperable, allows for a different level of research because the volume, speed, and variety of collected information makes it easier to generate scientific evidence with applications in medicine and other areas of health. Moreover, because information comes from different health systems (and from other sources), it is easy to understand the benefit in promoting global health which can benefit all people and not only those in more developed countries.

However, one of the problems associated with big data is the fact that its use is in the hands of private companies whose goal is not the common good but increased profits for shareholders, despite the acknowledged corporate social responsibility. In healthcare, the problem is even more complex because in many health systems, public hospital corporatization (Rego et al. 2010) and private modalities, such as the private finance initiative, are occurring. Therefore, the potential for misuse of these data is becoming an increasing concern for health authorities. Moreover, interconnectivity with insurance companies and pharmaceutical industries, namely in huge industrial conglomerates, may allow unlawful and unethical use of private information (Mayer-Schonberger and Ingelsson 2018).

In turn, the intersection between big data and artificial intelligence (AI), consisting of software and hardware systems that act in the physical or digital dimensions, seems to be inevitable in global economic development and thus, presents the problem in new terms (Schwab 2015). Indeed, the challenge of AI systems in health both in healthcare delivery and in public health is paramount (Househ et al. 2017). It may be of use in promoting new treatment modalities besides preventing life-threatening diseases. Indeed, it may provide clinicians with a more accurate and detailed analysis by helping with the diagnosis and treatment of many diseases. Further, it may be helpful for assisting caregivers in support of the elderly. Further, it may be extremely useful for real-time monitoring of patients, sometimes at long distances. From a global health perspective, AI can be instrumental in disease detection and in the development of new pharmaceuticals (Shachar et al. 2020). AI also has the potential to be of use in precision medicine and personalized healthcare.

The enormous potential of AI and its associated risks entail caution in its use. According to the Independent High-Level Expert Group on Artificial Intelligence (2019), all societies globally should use AI based on several guidelines:

1   Develop, deploy, and use AI systems in a way that adheres to the ethical principles of respect for human autonomy, prevention of harm, fairness, and explicability.
2   Pay particular attention to situations involving more vulnerable groups such as children, persons with disabilities, and others that have historically been disadvantaged or are at risk of exclusion, and to situations that are characterized by asymmetries of power or information, such as between employers and workers or between businesses and consumers.
3   Acknowledge that while bringing substantial benefits to individuals and society, AI systems may also pose certain risks and have a negative impact, including impacts which may be difficult to anticipate, identify, and/or measure (such as democracy, the rule of law, and distributive justice or on the human mind itself).
4   Ensure that the development, deployment, and use of AI systems meets the seven key requirements for trustworthy AI: (a) human agency and oversight; (b) technical robustness and safety; (c) privacy and data governance; (d) transparency; (e) diversity, nondiscrimination, and fairness; (f) environmental and societal well-being; and (g) accountability.
5   Foster research and innovation to help assess AI systems and to further the achievement of the requirements, disseminate results, open questions to the wider public, and systematically train a new generation of experts in AI ethics.
6   Involve stakeholders throughout the AI system life cycle. Foster training and education so that all stakeholders are aware of and trained in trustworthy AI.

A fair and accountable use of AI in global health therefore implies robust ethical data governance (European Union Agency for Fundamental Rights 2018).

ICT and Personal Privacy

Undoubtedly, in e-health, the right to privacy and confidentiality of data implies the strict compliance of professional secrecy by all agents involved in the processing of personal data as well as the scrupulous collecting and storing of electronic medical records, regardless of the format (conventional or digital). However, the generalization of health-related ICTs raises complex ethical and legal concerns.

An effective regulatory framework to safeguard the interests of users must exist. For example, the generalization of electronic medical records and their dissemination throughout the health intranet should be properly supervised by competent regulatory authorities.

In fact, in civilized societies, individual privacy is an especially protected value and can be only disturbed by reason of force majeure. Those responsible for the treatment of health information should take appropriate measures to protect confidentiality, ensure the safety of facilities and equipment, and control access to information along with reinforcing the duty of confidentiality and ethical education of all professionals. Further, healthcare services must prevent third parties from unduly accessing electronic medical records and computer systems containing health information, including their backup copies. This type of caution can ensure appropriate levels of security and fulfill the requirements established by the legislation that regulates the protection of personal data to prevent its destruction, alteration, dissemination, unauthorized access, or any other form of illicit treatment of information (European Union 1995). This process obviously implies that electronic medical records can only be consulted by the doctor in charge of the provision of healthcare to the person concerned or by another healthcare professional who is under the supervision of the doctor in charge, is bound by secrecy, and is able to only access the information that is strictly necessary.

However, the interface between privacy and autonomy also determines the universally recognized right of patients to be able to access medical information that directly concerns them. In some contexts, medical and health information have been differentiated. If health information allows for understanding all types of personal information (directly or indirectly linked to the present or future health of the individual, besides their clinical and family history), this concept then includes information intended to be used in health-related care that is medical information in the strictest sense. However, when personal information is defined by any information of any nature and in any format (including sound and images) relating to an identified or identifiable person (data subject), the question of the actual ownership of health information and of the clinical data recorded needs to be carefully considered.

Thus, the digitalization of the electronic medical record is an important measure for the modernization of the health system. However, it must be accompanied by the necessary precautions, so that the right to privacy is not violated in any way. The creation of information networks is an important achievement by the modern civilization since it allows access to information and sharing by previously excluded population strata. However, implementation of an intranet, which is an information network within a healthcare facility or the entire health system, may jeopardize the right to individual privacy. Measures should be implemented to limit unauthorized access to inside information. A possible solution for minimizing this problem is the implementation of protection mechanisms while accessing computer data, namely, by creating complex keywords at different levels that limit access to the patient, their family (with consent), or healthcare personnel directly associated with the patient. This can help reverse the current paradigm of unlimited access in which control is only performed by the access registry.

If the right of any citizen to be adequately informed about the disease is now recognized, then it can also be argued that the citizen has the right not to know about their health. This is because autonomy may contemplate exceptions to the doctrine of express consent (if this is the real will of the patient). Knowledge of personal genetic information or serology for human immunodeficiency virus (HIV) is paradigmatic example of this *right not to know* (as an expression of the right to self-determination and the right to identity and individuality). There may be circumstances in which, considering the ethical principle of non-maleficence, the healthcare professional must refrain from informing the patient if this is the patient's express wish. Excessive and/or unwanted information can clearly be harmful to the patient. For this reason, healthcare professionals frequently communicate information to the family. In this way, the right to self-determination is being respected. In the context of the implementation of informed consent, it is also important to mention the importance of the right to privacy. Self-determination aims to restrict any external intrusion, assuming no interference into the intimate sphere of the individual. The term *privacy* can encompass four different precepts (Reich 1999):

1   Physical privacy refers to limited physical accessibility, meaning the *right to be left alone*. This concept is adjacent to *physical integrity*.
2   Mental privacy refers to freedom in the plane of psychological intrusion, obtained through the restriction of manipulative interferences of the individual will. This helps prevent torture practices involving mind manipulation.
3   Decisional privacy refers to freedom of procedural interference, that is, the exclusion of third parties in the decision process. This concept has been invoked in the context of the lawfulness of voluntary termination of pregnancy up to the limit of fetal viability.
4   Informational privacy is achieved by imposing limits on unauthorized access to personal information and data of an individual nature, for example, test results for HIV or individual genetic data. It is one of the pillars of the duty of professional secrecy.

The privacy and confidentiality of health data imply the strict observance of professional secrecy by all agents involved in the processing of personal, biological, and/or genetic data, besides the scrupulous storage of the individual clinical process, whether in conventional or dematerialized format. The generalization of health information systems also raises complex ethical/legal concerns. There must be an effective regulatory framework to safeguard individual interests (Newman 2015).

However, it has been questioned whether this right to privacy is unlimited, that is, whether there are limits to the duty of secrecy and the deontological (and legal) rule of professional confidentiality. Although limited, the main objection to the breach of professional secrecy by healthcare professionals, along with individual privacy (which is a value and a right in itself), is the negative reflection that this attitude has on the internal morality of medicine and of other professions besides the way that these areas are socially viewed. In fact, if the doctor is allowed to disclose information about the patient even in a limited way, this limited disclosure does not guarantee the ordinary citizen that these limits cannot be arbitrarily dilated. Thus, a consequentialist argument must also be considered since it is within the general interest that the confidentiality of the clinical act be preserved within established ethical limits.

Individual privacy is a particularly protected value and can only be disturbed by reasons of force majeure, such as the legitimate interest of direct relatives in accessing genetic information of the index case and only if this information allows for determination of their own genetic status. Other cases where legitimacy is recognized and it is rather the duty of the health professional to break confidentiality refers to the proven existence of legitimate interests of third parties, including family members at risk of contracting contagious diseases, such as HIV, human papilloma virus (HPV), hepatitis, and tuberculosis, or situations of child abuse and neglect.

In this ethical-social context, citizens may not comprehend and accept that their personal data is used for purposes other than those declared. Progressively, the *principle of purpose limitation* must be respected. If personal data are obtained for a particular purpose, they should be used for a different purpose only in exceptional cases and those of real public relevance, for example, the use of clinical data for research purposes even though the data are anonymized (Mayer-Schönberger 2009). Otherwise, a new basic right may be set up soon, termed the *right to be forgotten*, that seeks to eliminate any information concerning the patient from the healthcare information systems, if this is the patient's expressed and consistent wish (Ausloos 2012; Correia et al. 2021). Indeed, the loss of control over personal data has fueled the debate in Europe and in the United States about the existence and limits of the *right to be forgotten* (Ambrose 2014; Bode and Jones 2017).

The collection, treatment, and dissemination of information by new technologies may endanger personal privacy, particularly in the face of indiscriminate access through ICTs. A universal awareness, in which this loss of control over personal data is not acceptable, has now emerged with the view of strengthening individual rights. This awareness is the reason why the General Data Protection Regulation (GDPR) (European Union 2016) has suggested a new full *right to erasure* (Article 17 of the GDPR) by complying with certain requirements:

1   The data are no longer required in view of the purpose for which they were collected or processed.
2   The data subject withdraws consent.
3   The data subject opposes to processing and there are no legitimate grounds for denying this request.
4   The data were processed illegally.

Thus, there is a radical paradigm shift in healthcare delivery, namely in the inter-face between digital health and the right to privacy. This interface lacks the imple-mentation of guidelines that guarantee the protection of these rights. Healthcare regulators and the international community should play a central role, given their special responsibility to protect the basic rights of citizens (Ahmed 2017).

Conclusion

Global health is a worthwhile goal for different reasons. First, health is an essential good for the human condition. We must promote it universally so that all human beings can enjoy this right. Indeed, most developed societies recognize the exist-ence of a basic right of access to healthcare of appropriate quality and consider it a positive welfare right (Nunes et al. 2017). Second, global health is important because globalization has allowed us to approach different people by stimulating interconnectivity, for example, through social networking. This implies that social and economic inequalities among people and even within each society are pro-gressively less tolerated. Third, even in the absence of truly effective institutions of global governance, interdependence has become the keyword regarding relations between peoples (Jia and Wang 2019). Therefore, global health presents a win-win situation for all concerned parties.

This implies that if no policy exists, there is at least a global vision of health, as described by the SDGs (GBD 2017; SDG Collaborators 2018). Besides LMICs, health literacy is paramount in wealthy nations as well (Oni et al. 2019). A health literacy program that draws attention to the importance of cross-sectoral efforts should include other areas, such as education, economics, and/or agriculture, and should enroll younger generations. Indeed, young people want to be involved in actively achieving the SDGs and especially a fair global health system (Bulc et al. 2019). Engaging all young people is essential in the design and delivery of global public goods, such as health and social well-being, while considering their diverse backgrounds. Further, global health, environmental protection, and addressing climate change are part of our common humanitarian endeavor and one of the most important opportunities in the upcoming decades (Capon and Corvalana 2018).

Global health, however, will face new challenges, namely the digital economy and e-health. AI may be an appropriate tool to address some of the obstacles to its universal implementation (World Health Organization 2019). Further, global health must be implemented in a variable economic and political geometry, with many low-income countries being failed states that are still very far away from advanced democracies. The political and demographic consequences of this global imbalance is yet to be evaluated.

References

Ahmed W. 2017. The ethics of memory in a digital age: Interrogating the right to be forgot-ten. *Information Communication & Society* 20 (12): 1833–1833.

Ambrose ML. 2014. Speaking of forgetting: Analysis of possible non-EU responses to the right to be forgotten and speech exception. *Telecommunications Policy* 38 (8–9): 800–811. DOI: 10.1016/j.telpol.2014.05.002.

American Medical Association. 2019. Professionalism in the use of social media. www.ama-assn.org/delivering-care/ethics/professionalism-use-social-media.

American Telemedicine Association. 2019. www.americantelemed.org/.

Ausloos J. 2012. The "right to be forgotten" – Worth remembering? *Computer Law & Security Review* 28 (2): 143–152.

Bode L and Jones ML. 2017. Ready to forget: American attitudes toward the right to be forgotten. *Information Society* 33 (2): 76–85. DOI: 10.1080/01972243.2016.1271071.

Boman M and Kruse E. 2017. Supporting global health goals with information and communications technology. *Global Health Action* 10 (3): 6–13.

Bulc B, Al-Wahdani B, Bustreo F et al. 2019. Urgency for transformation: Youth engagement in global health. *The Lancet* 7: 1–2.

Campos J, Sharma P, Gabiria UG et al. 2017. A big data analytical architecture for the asset management. *Procedia CIRP* 64: 369–374.

Capon A and Corvalana C. 2018. Climate change and health: Global issue, local responses. *Public Health Research & Practice* 28 (4): 1–3.

Correia M, Rego G and Nunes R. 2021. Gender transition: Is there a right to be forgotten. *Health Care Analysis*. https://doi.org/10.1007/s10728-021-00433-1.

Drosou M, Jagadish HV, Pitoura E et al. 2017. Diversity in big data: A review. *Big Data* 5: 73–84.

Engebretsen E and Heggen K. 2015. Powerful concepts in global health. Comment on "Knowledge, moral claims and the exercise of power in global health". *International Journal of Health Policy and Management* 4 (2): 115–117.

European Parliament. 2011. Directive 2011/24/EU of the European parliament and of the council of 9 March 2011 on the application of patients' rights in cross-border healthcare. https://eur-lex.europa.eu/legal-content/EN/TXT/?uri=CELEX%3A32011L0024.

European Union. 1995. The data protection directive. Directive 95/46/EC of the European parliament and of the council of 24 October 1995 on the protection of individuals with regard to the processing of personal data and on the free movement of such data. http://eur-lex.europa.eu/legal-content/PT/TXT/?uri=LEGISSUM:l14012.

European Union. 2016. General data protection regulation. Regulation (EU) 2016/679 of the European parliament and of the council of 27 April 2016 on the protection of natural persons with regard to the processing of personal data and on the free movement of such data. http://eur-lex.europa.eu/legal-content/PT/TXT/?uri=CELEX:32016R0679.

European Union Agency for Fundamental Rights. 2018. BigData: Discrimination in data-supported decision making. http://fra.europa.eu/en/publication/2018/big-data-discrimination.

GBD 2016 Lifetime Risk of Stroke Collaborators. 2018. Global, regional, and country-specific lifetime risks of stroke, 1990 and 2016. *New England Journal of Medicine* 379 (25): 2429–2437.

GBD 2017 Mortality Collaborators. 2018. Global, regional, and national age-sex-specific mortality and life expectancy, 1950–2017: A systematic analysis for the global burden of disease study 2017. *The Lancet* 392: 1684–1735.

GBD 2017 SDG Collaborators. 2018. Measuring progress from 1990 to 2017 and projecting attainment to 2030 of the health-related sustainable development goals for 195 countries and territories: A systematic analysis for the global burden of disease study 2017. *The Lancet* 392: 2091–2138.

Househ MS, Aldosari B, Alanazi A et al. 2017. Big data, big problems: A healthcare perspective. *Studies in Health, Technology and Informatics* 238: 36–39.

Ienca M, Ferretti A, Hurst S et al. 2018. Considerations for ethics review of big data health research: A scoping review. *PloS One*, 13, e0204937.

Independent High-Level Expert Group on Artificial Intelligence set up by the European Commission. 2019. Ethics guidelines for trustworthy AI. European Commission, Brussels, Document made public on 8 April 2019.

Jia P and Wang Y. 2019. Global health efforts and opportunities related to the belt and road initiative. *The Lancet* 7: 703–705.

Kaebnick G and Gusmano M. 2019. Forget about "because science". Persuading people to vaccinate their children requires engaging with them about their values. Slate. https://slate.com/technology/2019/04/vaccination-values-science-based-policy.html.

Kaslow D. 2018. Vaccine candidates for poor nations are going to waste. *Nature* 564: 337–339.

Kayaalp M. 2017. Patient privacy in the era of big data. *Balkan Medical Journal.* DOI: 10.4274/balkanmedj.2017.0966.

Koplan JP, Bond TC, Merson MH et al. 2009. Towards a common definition of global health. *The Lancet* 373 (9679): 1993–1995.

Mayer-Schönberger V. 2009. *Delete: The virtue of forgetting in the digital age.* Princeton University Press, Princeton.

Mayer-Schonberger V and Ingelsson E. 2018. Big data and medicine: A big deal? *Journal of Internal Medicine* 283: 418–429.

McLuhan M and Powers B. 1989. *Chapter 1: The resonating interval in the global village. Transformations in world life and media in the 21st century.* Oxford University Press, Oxford.

Mittelstadt BD and Floridi L. 2016. The ethics of big data: Current and foreseeable issues in biomedical contexts. *Science and Engineering Ethics* 22 (2): 303–341. DOI: 10.1007/s11948-015-9652-2.

Newman AL. 2015. What the "right to be forgotten" means for privacy in a digital age. *Science* 347 (6221): 507–508.

Nunes R. 2020. Addressing gender inequality to promote basic human rights and development: A global perspective. CEDIS Working Papers 2020 (1). ISBN: 978-989-54596-2-9.

Nunes R, Nunes SB and Rego G. 2017. Healthcare as a universal right. *Journal of Public Health* 25: 1–9.

Nunes R and Rego G. 2014. Priority setting in health care: A complementary approach. *Health Care Analysis* 22: 292–303.

Oni T, Yudkin J, Fonn S et al. 2019. Global public health starts at home: Upstream approaches to global health training. *The Lancet* 7: 301–302.

Rego G, Nunes R and Costa J. 2010. The challenge of corporatisation: The experience of Portuguese public hospitals. *The European Journal of Health Economics* 1 (4): 367–381.

Reich WT. 1999. *Encyclopedia of bioethics.* Simon & Schuster and Prentice Hall International, London.

Schwab K. 2015. *The fourth industrial revolution.* Foreign Affairs. www.foreignaffairs.com/articles/2015-12-12/fourth-industrial-revolution [Accessed 29 November 2021].

Sen A. 1999. *Development as freedom.* Knopf, New York.

Shachar C, Gerke S and Adashi E. 2020. AI surveillance during pandemics: Ethical implementation imperatives. *The Hastings Center Report* 50 (3): 18–21.

Taylor R and Alper J. 2018. Using technology to advance global health. Proceedings of a workshop. Forum on Public-Private Partnerships for Global Health and Safety. Board on Global Health. Health and Medicine Division. The National Academies Press, Washington DC.

Terrasse M, Gorin M and Sisti D. 2019. Social media, e-health, and medical ethics. *The Hastings Center Report* 49 (1): 24–33.

United Nations. 2021. Sustainable development goals. www.un.org/sustainabledevelopment/ sustainable-development-goals/.

World Health Organization. 2019. *WHO guideline recommendations on digital interventions for health system strengthening.* World Health Organization, Genève. License: CC BY-NC-SA 3.0 IGO. www.who.int/en/.

World Health Organization. 2021. *Thirteenth programme of work 2019-2023.* World Health Organization, Genève. https://www.who.int/en/

7 COVID-19 and Global Public Goods

The recent coronavirus pandemic (SARS-CoV-2) and the associated disease, COVID-19, implies a rethinking of global ethics. The universal system of fundamental rights developed over the 20th century, which affirms the identity of the human being and the uniqueness of the person, has had a limited impact on uniting different peoples for diverse geopolitical reasons. Indeed, in a realistic view of international relations, different sovereign states' exercise of power was the decisive element in the conduct of relations between different nations, with economic globalization being merely instrumental and inconsequential in terms of the application of universal ethics. Indeed, it has not yet been possible to develop true planetary ethics.

It is certain, however, that economic globalization has resulted in an improvement in the living conditions of hundreds of millions of people, reducing world poverty considerably over the past decades (The World Bank Group 2018). Therefore, the enjoyment of social and economic rights was indirectly promoted (Nunes 2020). Today, many more people around the world have access to health services or quality education systems.

However, this positive externality of economic globalization was not accompanied by the construction of a true planetary awareness about the need for a common humanitarianism that is genuine and centered on the essentiality of the person and their dignity. The COVID-19 pandemic should alert us to the need for broad ontological solidarity among all people to join efforts to overcome global problems that need global responses. Without a global ethics that unifies different people and stimulates the best that exists in each other, humanity can hardly respond to this pandemic, to future pandemics that will surely arise, to pressing environmental and climatic problems, and to growing migratory phenomena, among many other global challenges (Kovacevic and Jahic 2020).

Even though health is a very personal experience, it is also a global phenomenon since we are facing a pandemic with important global health repercussions (Oni et al. 2019). The purpose of this chapter is to suggest the need for robust healthcare systems to face the pandemic and contribute to a growing awareness of the need for true global public goods such as health, health education, and universal access to COVID-19 vaccination. In addition, I propose legally binding instruments to accomplish this goal.

DOI: 10.4324/9781003241065-8

Medicine, Public Health, and the Health System

Never since World War II has humanity faced a global challenge such as the COVID-19 pandemic. It has been a challenge for patients, healthcare professionals, and society at large. As a global uncontrolled phenomenon and a public health emergency, the first response was to temporarily uphold basic liberties and fundamental rights through the approval of specific legislation that empowers governments to do so. Even in advanced democracies, basic liberties were upheld to contain the spread of the virus. Immediately, all over the world, travel restrictions within a country and between countries were implemented, including quarantine and mass testing of travelers and lockdowns of countries, regions, and cities was the norm. Cordon sanitaire and mass quarantine were regular practices. Further, strict physical distancing between citizens with the goal of flattening the epidemic curve and controlling the pandemic was imposed (Gostin et al. 2020).

However, balancing public health with civil liberties also meant closing public spaces (schools, childcare, workplaces, and mass transit) everywhere, sometimes without a clear rationale, and draconian measures, for instance, in nursing homes that restricted residents from leaving or visitors from entering the facilities. However, the Nuffield Council on Bioethics (2020) suggested that

> People should be treated as moral equals, worthy of respect. While individuals may be asked to make sacrifices for the public good, the respect due to individuals should never be forgotten in the way in which interventions such as quarantine and self-isolation are implemented.

The psychological impact of these measures is yet to be fully determined. However, it is now clear that social separation frequently leads to loneliness, emotional detachment, and even a disruption of social life. In addition, family bonding and social connectedness have been disrupted, namely regarding the elderly who became even more isolated and the youngsters who saw their social life postponed for a long time. COVID-19 had another dramatic effect: family clustering. This is a confirmed phenomenon associated with this pandemic because all families are crushed by disease, with multiple cases of death, hospitalization, quarantine, or social distancing in nursing homes. Thus, the least restrictive means necessary to accomplish the public health goal should be implemented because civil liberties and human rights cannot be suspended even when facing this pandemic.

It is true that the healthcare system will only respond adequately after flattening the pandemic curve and therefore, save lives. Meanwhile, to fight the coronavirus (SARS-CoV-2) pandemic appropriately, the existence of a well-funded and well-structured universal public health system is of fundamental importance. The countries that best responded to this crisis were also those that had universal access to quality and timely care for the entire population. In contrast, less structured systems with a low level of funding quickly became overcrowded with professional exhaustion and a high mortality rate. However, the coronavirus pandemic has not only questioned the health system's response to patients especially vulnerable to the disease but also questioned the delivery of healthcare to the general population as well (Wang and Volkow 2021). Indeed, no system was prepared for such a huge and concentrated demand for healthcare. No system had enough critical care beds, ventilators, medicines, and personal protective equipment (such as masks) considering that an estimated 2% of all COVID-19 patients may require ventilators.

In addition, this pandemic was a huge challenge for healthcare professionals. Nevertheless, in most societies, respect for the patient and compliance with ethical principles and professional guidelines was the usual practice. Even when facing scarcity of resources, physicians always considered valuing the patient and not exclusively the disease, including perception of its severity. In addition, equality and nondiscrimination due to characteristics such as nationality, gender, ethnicity, and chronological age were the main ethical drivers of healthcare professionals. For instance, in none of the cases, age alone was the only element considered in the prioritization strategies.

In the clinical setting, sharing the decision-making process between the healthcare team, the patient, and the family with honest and transparent communication among all, given the extraordinary nature of the situation, was fundamental, especially in the admission to intensive care (Rosenbaum 2020). To ensure a resilient and diligent practice means the existence of clear, explicit, and transparent criteria for prioritizing and admitting patients to intensive care, such that:

1   The criteria must be consensual, approved by representative professional associations, and universally implemented.
2   In the face of scarcity of resources and the impossibility of admitting all patients in need of intensive care, the guideline should be maximizing survival until hospital discharge, the number of years of life saved, or the possibilities of living at each stage of life.
3   Special attention should be paid to critical and unstable patients who need intensive monitoring and treatment that cannot be provided outside an intensive care unit.
4   The opportunity cost principle must be considered: admitting one patient may imply denying another admission; therefore, as an absolute rule, the criterion *first to arrive first* must be avoided.
5   In a situation of absolute scarcity of resources and equipment, admitting people for whom a minimum benefit is expected should be considered, such as situations of established multiorgan failure, high risk of death calculated by severity scales, very limited functional situations, or conditions of very advanced fragility.

These criteria should be applied uniformly to all people and hospitals and not selectively to the elderly or patients with chronic pathologies. Monitoring the application of these criteria by regulatory authorities as well as supervising the enjoyment of non-COVID patients' rights are paramount. Therefore, it is important to design ethical criteria for admission to treatment, namely in an environment with scarce resources (Emanuel et al. 2020), for both patients with and without COVID-19. In fact, the COVID-19 pandemic posed the question of establishing ethical criteria for admission to intensive care, innovative medicines, or even an effective vaccination. This means that although there is sufficient installed capacity for assisted ventilation, in ordinary circumstances, conditions should exist for the purchase of an appreciable amount of equipment to anticipate future needs in a more unfavorable scenario.

Moreover, this pandemic showed the need for adequate planning of psychological support actions for patients, families, and professionals, given the emotional impact and moral distress of highly complex ethical decisions. Indeed, burnout is common among professionals, particularly when complex moral dilemmas are at stake. During the COVID-19 pandemic, healthcare professionals have had a high workload and have been exposed to multiple psychosocial stressors on personal and work- and client-related settings (Duarte et al. 2020).

In short, the COVID-19 pandemic questioned old paradigms of action and recalled a set of policy issues that need differentiated approaches on a global scale:

1   Decision based on data and scientific evidence;
2   Access to health, particularly the rights of the elderly, minorities, and people with disabilities;
3   Establishment of priorities in healthcare access and fairness in the allocation of resources;
4   Consent for compulsive treatment;
5   Limitation on access to health for non-COVID patients;
6   Telemedicine and e-health;
7   Ethics and mental health;
8   Women's and children's health, and reproductive health;
9   Gender equality and COVID-19;
10   Death and dying during the pandemic;
11   Privacy of positive health professionals, working conditions, and protection;
12   Hospital collaboration between public and private sectors.

In a public health emergency, science and evidence are necessary in all aspects of public policy. For instance, if it is not possible to test and treat everyone, how can we determine who should be tested and who should be vaccinated? Scarce evidence suggests the need to protect high-risk people, such as the elderly, or prioritizing those that are in confined settings such as nursing homes. In addition, patients with underlying conditions, such as heart or lung disease and diabetes, should be tested and vaccinated first as to their mortality rate associated with COVID-19 is higher. Meanwhile, protecting critical services such as healthcare professionals, public safety, and fire protection workers was also deemed an adequate measure worldwide.

These choices are particularly meaningful because there is now robust evidence on the transmission of COVID-19 by asymptomatic carriers (Camilla et al. 2020). In addition, there is evidence on person-to-person transmission during the incubation period (Yu et al. 2020). Since the PCR test is highly specific and sensitive to the COVID-19 genome but can yield negative results, it should be acknowledged that such patients are contagious and may develop infection because they are false negative for virus or are still in a window of negativity (Corman et al. 2020). A decision based on data and scientific evidence is, of course, one of the issues to consider.

However, this pandemic also showed that the lack of scientific evidence allowed the arbitrary use of available medicines in many countries worldwide. From a medical perspective, however, it is important to implement measures to identify patients at risk of overmedication or iatrogenic intervention, protecting them from disproportionate medical invasion, namely from therapeutic innovation, and suggesting medical interventions that are ethically and clinically acceptable (Vogt et al. 2016). Indeed, doubts remain regarding the therapeutic effectiveness of remdesivir and hydroxychloroquine.

To promote health, prevent disease, and restore health, a distinction is classically made between primordial, primary, secondary, and tertiary prevention. On the one hand, interventions with broad social and economic reach that, by themselves, affect the health of a population. Policies promoting healthy lifestyles, such as prevention of smoking, drug addiction, alcoholism, or the use of masks and social etiquette, fall within this concept of primordial prevention. On the other hand, primary prevention targets individuals or the general population and aims to reduce the incidence of the disease. COVID-19 vaccination or health education are concrete examples of this type of social prevention. Secondary prevention uses, for example, screening for a disease (COVID-19 mass testing) to detect the disease early, with important impacts on its prevalence and associated morbidity and mortality. Tertiary prevention aims to limit the development of a disease, prevent or minimize its complications, and promote family, social, and even labor reintegration. Quaternary prevention aims to reduce the risk of iatrogenic and inappropriate use of medications. It is a model in which 4P medicine (predictive, preventive, participated, and personalized) combines the different existing technological resources to obtain the best health outcomes. COVID-19 is a good example of how 4P medicine can be socially and individually useful.

The limitation of access to healthcare for non-COVID-19 patients was also a major problem worldwide, with increasing mortality rates associated with diseases other than COVID-19. Indeed, the healthcare system must guarantee the basic rights of citizens. That is, health is a fundamental value in any society; therefore, there is a clear need to prevent practices of unjustified discrimination of patients. This practice should be regarded as a dysfunction of the healthcare system during the pandemic. Cream-skimming practices may occur when the provider (the physician or other professional) or even the hospital discriminates against patients (individuals or groups of patients) because COVID-19 patients are prioritized. Although cream-skimming is often at stake in the healthcare sector, it is important to avoid unethical discrimination of patients because all patients matter, not just COVID-19 ones.

Indeed, elective procedures were upheld in all countries during the pandemic, whether intentionally or indirectly, because all efforts were focused on the management of the pandemics. All healthcare systems called for curtailing nonessential adult and child nonelective medical and surgical procedures with the intent of flattening the curve. According to Bodilsen et al. (2021)

> Hospital admissions for all major non-covid-19 disease groups decreased during national lockdowns compared with the pre-pandemic baseline period. Additionally, mortality rates were higher overall and for patients admitted to hospital with conditions such as respiratory diseases, cancer, pneumonia, and sepsis.

Considering that discrimination against non-COVID patients may be intersectional, meaning that not only the disease but also the existence of disability, gender, ethnicity, etc. may contribute to discrimination, measures should be taken to avoid this practice. This is especially regarding gender discrimination because it is well known that existing disparities were aggravated during the pandemics, namely regarding access to reproductive technologies or procedures instrumental to the right not to reproduce, such as abortion or tubal ligations.

Human Rights and Public Goods

The COVID-19 pandemic has had a paradoxical effect on most countries. On the one hand, the need to protect human rights was emphasized, namely the right to access healthcare, nondiscrimination, and protection of privacy. On the other hand, since this is a very serious public health problem, restrictive measures of human rights were implemented in accordance with the collective interest from a utilitarian perspective of the pursuit of public interest. There were two main drivers: first, to flatten the pandemic curve and therefore, reduce the pressure on the healthcare system. Second, to achieve robust community protection from COVID-19. For a country to reach herd immunity, 80% to 85% of the population needs to be vaccinated. Therefore, improving vaccination rates will require adequate planning and a strategic delivery plan.

As we are only safe when the most vulnerable among us are safe, the major principles of public health were universally applied, namely rigorous contact tracing, accurate diagnosis, and quarantine. Surveillance modes, such as thermal scanners or web cameras (including facial recognition), were commonly used. Mass testing (PCR, antigen, and antibody), sequencing for new mutations of SARS-CoV-2, and vaccination were used to prevent further spread of the virus. Frequently, digital contact tracing using mobile technology was used (Martinez-Martin et al. 2020) to reopen countries, assuming that a healthy nation is an economic nation.

Indeed, the implementation of the following measures was common practice:

1   Compulsory social distancing;
2   Compulsory public health measures, such as quarantine, lockdown, wearing a mask, and mandatory vaccination;

3 Digital contact tracing systems;
4 Digitalization of health;
5 Strategies for herd immunity;
6 Corona Passport/COVID Certificate and movement limitation;
7 Clinical trials of drugs for COVID-19 and exposure of participants to the virus;
8 Rationing of vaccines and selection of priority groups (health professionals, security forces, vulnerable populations, etc.); and
9 Community ethics and duty of assistance.

During the pandemic, the intersection between human rights and public interest has resulted in important conflicts, generating social concern in many civilized countries. Privacy and autonomy protection was a challenge in many countries, for instance, regarding digital contact tracing systems. In addition, public health measures such as compulsory social distancing led to increased rates of suicide, family and gender violence, and individualist behavior. Movement limitation, for instance, through the implementation of the Corona Passport, the COVID Certificate in the European Union (EU) (European Commission 2021), with or without facial recognition was also a disputed initiative. This is because individual privacy, equity, and a balance between developed and underdeveloped countries was also at stake.

The COVID-19 pandemic also showed that the pattern of economic globalization must evolve to a more balanced structure because it is difficult to accept that most countries became hostages of a few economies. For instance, the world distribution of high-tech technologies such as respirators, masks, and gloves must be revisited. In addition, the production and distribution of pharmaceuticals was a major issue in the COVID-19 pandemic due to a lack of scientific evidence and a global capacity for distribution.

It is therefore necessary, from a global public health perspective, that the World Health Organization (WHO) and other institutions such as the United Nations Economic, Social, and Cultural Organization (UNESCO) have a prior role in generating scientific evidence and in planetary cooperation in knowledge sharing. This is especially regarding the investigation of new drugs for the treatment of diseases, in the search for a vaccination of universal application, or even contributing to health literacy and basic measures of social hygiene, such as the use of masks, the measurement of body temperature, or the way in which people should cough or sneeze in public (Bulc et al. 2019).

Nonscientifically validated therapies can be used exceptionally and compassionately if there is no alternative medication that has been sifted through evidence-based medicine. However, this should be always with strict medical and international health authorities' monitoring and without placing false expectations on the population. However, only randomized clinical trials can prove the real benefits of innovative therapies. For example, Dexamethasone has shown therapeutic benefits in the treatment of COVID-19. However, remdesivir and especially hydroxychloroquine have shown questionable benefit, although they are used frequently in some countries. Hence, there is a need for coordinated international strategy to present clear information to the populations in an impartial way and without undue influences from social and political actors in this complex matter.

As an example of measures of general interest and considering that a single country cannot manage global public health, the European Commission suggested the creation of a European Union for Health involving the 27 states of the union. The central objectives were linked to the need to increase the capacity to respond to new global crises, such as the COVID-19 pandemic, the creation of conditions for less dependence on other countries, creating a strategic reserve of medicines, and implementing supranational health policies. This proposal is, moreover, in the wake of the central values of modern democracies. For example, the draft European Constitutional Treaty foresaw the right to health protection as a basic right of European citizenship. More recently, the EU Directive, which establishes the rules for access to cross-border healthcare and promotes cooperation in health between different countries, corresponds to the EU's strategic orientation (European Parliament 2011).

Assuming that each member state has already organized a universal healthcare system, how can these ideals be realized? First, there should be promotion of the articulation and the integration of the different health systems and harmonizing procedures so that there is a decentralized integration of health. That is, coordination at the European level and administration at the national or regional level. Digital health, that is, the use of the most modern information and communication technologies, will be an essential tool to guarantee the interoperability and interconnectivity of the health systems of the different member states of the union (Independent High-Level Expert Group on Artificial Intelligence 2019).

However, it is necessary to strategically implement a genuine EU health policy. This is because private transnational companies oversee the production of new drugs, sometimes even large industrial conglomerates. This implies that states alone experience difficulty in negotiating prices and creating strategic reserves. It is clear, for reasons of scale, that the EU has the means to create this strategic reserve. Finally, if there is an area where cooperation between different states is imperative, it is in terms of global health (United Nations 2020). That is, public health problems may not concern an individual state, but they need articulated responses at the regional or even global level. Therefore, it is essential to reinforce the competences of the European Centre for Disease Prevention and Control and to stimulate the creation of innovative centers in biotechnology. Therefore, the European Union for Health is a huge step toward the implementation of the social welfare model, providing citizens with greater protection in access to health. This example can be followed on a planetary scale if we want global justice to succeed.

This implies the adoption of a different ethics on behalf of people, and therefore, the use of medicine, health technologies, and modern information and communication technologies (including artificial intelligence (AI), quantum computing, and the treatment of big data) according to principles of justice and equity, of centralization in the sick person and in their quality of life, and in the protection of essential civilizational values, such as respect for individual privacy (European Union 2016). However, imperative reasons for global public health may, transiently and justifiably, in a proportional manner and with a concrete purpose originate a different course of action. For example, AI has been used with enormous success in China and Canada for contact tracing, that is, to identify all people (contacts) who have been exposed to respiratory droplets or secretions from a COVID-19 case. Undoubtedly, contact tracing using AI is more effective than manual tracking, thus allowing the stratification of the risk of exposure and implementing measures such as prophylactic isolation or surveillance. Thus, AI can help prevent the spread of this infectious disease (Shachar et al. 2020).

As this was the first pandemic in the age of globalization strongly driven by the enormous mobility that exists today on a global scale, it also meant that institutions of global health governance, such as the WHO, found global solutions for global problems. This was mainly in terms of the information to be provided to citizens of different countries, in terms of risk of contagion, screening strategies, risk groups, circuits of circulation of patients in hospitals, mortality, and postinfection sequelae, among other fundamental information (World Health Organization 2020a).

The WHO is a world leader in the vaccination of children. It has helped decrease the global incidence of deaths from measles, polio, smallpox, and many other childhood diseases. Smallpox, for example, is now eradicated; since the 1970s, two hundred million children were vaccinated annually across the planet (World Health Organization 2019). Further, the WHO is still responsible for coordinating health policies on a global scale. In formulating concrete proposals, the WHO has proven to be essential in generating scientific evidence and disseminating best practices in this field. Otherwise, different countries would be at the mercy of erratic policies without a scientific basis, with great damage to the population. As a result, there is an enormous need for efficient international coordination with real power to facilitate effective cooperation on global health. As Chelsea Clinton (Clinton et al. 2020) says, the WHO "must be even more independent, collaborate with nongovernmental organizations, and increase the emphasis on human rights."

For instance, it should be determined whether COVID-19 vaccination should be mandatory to increase vaccination rates, or if values such as liberty and autonomy should imply a global campaign of health literacy and education showing people the benefit to individuals, families, and societies of getting all people vaccinated to protect the well-being of individuals or communities (World Health Organization 2021). However, vaccination should be considered a global public good. This means that efforts should be made to overcome the huge disparities in the global distribution of vaccines enrolling both international institutions and other international players such as private corporations, not-for-profit corporations, and even nongovernmental organizations. The international initiative to promote equitable access to vaccination, COVID-19 Vaccines Global Access (COVAX), enrolling partners such as coalition for epidemic preparedness innovations (CEPI), the vaccine alliance (GAVI), the world health organization (WHO), and the United Nations Children Fund (UNICEF), is an example of a coordinated international support for global health.

However, despite efforts at the regional level or by international organizations such as the WHO for humanity to pursue global public goods such as global health, an International Convention for Pandemics should be considered by competent global organizations. This legally binding instrument, according to international law, will be an essential step to consider global health as an essential global public good. This treaty should determine the ways of international cooperation, namely regarding universal vaccination. Indeed, global justice and solidarity cannot end with the COVID-19 pandemic and different global strategies must be implemented (Klugman 2020).

Conclusion

Nothing is the same after the coronavirus (SARS-CoV-2) pandemic. In this context, both biological and social Darwinism should be balanced with international efforts to promote global public goods. Thus, humanity together is prepared to respond to this type of phenomenon with humility, because if everyone is equal in the face of the threat, socioeconomic conditions (including ethnicity, gender, etc.) should also be considered (World Health Organization 2020b). What could be the responses in the face of a global pandemic?

First, ensuring high levels of health literacy is important so that local communities are more resilient to combat these threats. Protecting life and livelihood is essential because the spread of SARS-CoV-2 depends on personal and social habits. It should not be forgotten that the pandemic was associated with more child abuse, suicides, and drug overdoses. Nearly half percent of the deaths occurred in nursing homes. Therefore, combating poverty and establishing fair and appropriate health systems is also paramount.

However, the health systems will evolve dramatically in the coming years, for instance in primary care. This is because an impressive transformation has already occurred in response to the pandemic regarding the digital transition, and the generalization of digital systems and video consultation. Thus, promoting the implementation of robust healthcare systems and considering access to health as a universal human right should be a landmark in the post-pandemic era.

In addition, promoting scientific research worldwide to develop new medicines and vaccines to combat this threat is essential. This is because the effects of COVID-19 continue for weeks or months beyond the initial illness. Indeed, managing new or ongoing symptoms four weeks or more after the start of acute COVID-19 will be a challenge for most societies (NICE 2020). This *long COVID* should be managed with the best available evidence gathered internationally.

Finally, a fair balance between the developed and developing world, namely through international cooperation and strengthening international organizations such as the WHO, UNESCO, and UNICEF, should be reached. Further, the approval of an International Convention for Pandemics may be a huge step toward these goals.

References

Bodilsen J, Nielsen P, Søgaard M et al. 2021. Hospital admission and mortality rates for non-covid diseases in Denmark during covid-19 pandemic: Nationwide population based cohort study. *BMJ* 373: n1135. https://doi.org/10.1136/bmj.n1135.

Bulc B, Al-Wahdani B, Bustreo F et al. 2019. Urgency for transformation: Youth engagement in global health. *The Lancet* 7: 1–2.

Camilla R, Schunk M, Sothmann P et al. 2020. Transmission of 2019-nCoV infection from an asymptomatic contact in Germany. *New England Journal of Medicine* 382 (10): 970–971.

Clinton C, Friedman E, Gostin L and Sridhar D. 2020. Why the WHO? *Think Global Health*: 1–6. 5 June. www.thinkglobalhealth.org/article/why-who?utm_source=thinkglob alhealth&utm_medium=email&utm_campaign=New%20Campaign&utm_con tent=B&utm_term=TGH.

Corman V, Landt O, Kaiser M et al. 2020. Detection of 2019 novel coronavirus (2019-nCoV) by real-time RT-PCR. *Eurosurveillance* 5 (3): 23–30.

Duarte I, Teixeira A, Castro L et al. 2020. Burnout among Portuguese healthcare workers during the COVID-19 pandemic. *BMC Public Health* 20: 188520. https://doi.org/10.1186/s12889-020-09980-z.

Emanuel E, Persad G, Upshur R et al. 2020. Fair allocation of medical resources in the time of Covid-19. *The New England Journal of Medicine* 382: 2049–2055.

European Commission. 2021. Guidelines on paper version of the EU Digital COVID Certificate. eHealth Network, Brussels [Accessed 26 May 2021].

European Parliament. 2011. Directive 2011/24/EU of the European parliament and of the council of 9 March 2011 on the application of patients' rights in cross-border healthcare. https://eur-lex.europa.eu/legal-content/EN/TXT/?uri=CELEX%3A32011L0024.

European Union. 2016. General data protection regulation. Regulation (EU) 2016/679 of the European parliament and of the council of 27 April 2016 on the protection of natural persons with regard to the processing of personal data and on the free movement of such data. http://eur-lex.europa.eu/legal-content/PT/TXT/?uri=CELEX:32016R0679.

Gostin L, Friedman E, Wetter S. 2020. Responding to Covid-19: How to navigate a public health emergency legally and ethically. *The Hastings Center Report* 50 (2): 8–12.

Independent High-Level Expert Group on Artificial Intelligence set up by the European Commission. 2019. Ethics guidelines for trustworthy AI. European Commission, Brussels, Document made public on 8 April 2019.

Klugman K. 2020. Global solidarity can't end with the COVID-19 pandemic. *Think Global Health Newsletter*. 11 December.

Kovacevic M and Jahic A. 2020. COVID-19 and human development: Exploring global preparedness and vulnerability. *Human Development Data Story*. UNDP, New York 29 April.

Martinez-Martin N, Wieten S, Magnus D et al. 2020. Digital contact tracing, privacy, and public health. *The Hastings Center Report* 50 (3): 43–46.

NICE. 2020. COVID-19 rapid guideline: Managing the long-term effects of COVID-19, NICE guideline. *National Institute for Health and Care Excellence*. 18 December 2020 www.nice.org.uk/guidance/ng188.

Nuffield Council on Bioethics. 2020. *Ethical considerations in responding to the COVID-19 pandemic. Rapid policy briefing.* Nuffield Council on Bioethics, London. 17 March 2020.

Nunes R. 2020. Addressing gender inequality to promote basic human rights and development: A global perspective. *CEDIS Working Papers* 2020 (1). http://cedis.fd.unl.pt/

blog/project/addressing-gender-inequality-to-promote-basic-human-rights-and-development-a-global-perspective/.

Oni T, Yudkin J, Fonn S et al. 2019. Global public health starts at home: Upstream approaches to global health training. *The Lancet* 7: 301–302.

Rosenbaum L. 2020. Facing Covid-19 in Italy: Ethics, logistics, and therapeutics on the epidemic's front line. *New England Journal of Medicine Perspective*: 1–3. 18 March 2020.

Shachar C, Gerke S and Adashi E. 2020. AI surveillance during pandemics: Ethical implementation imperatives. *The Hastings Center Report* 50 (3): 18–21.

United Nations. 2020. Sustainable development goals. www.un.org/sustainabledevelopment/sustainable-development-goals/.

Vogt H, Hofmann B and Getz L. 2016. The new holism: P4 systems medicine and the medicalization of health and of life itself. *Medicine, Healthcare and Philosophy* 19: 307–323.

Wang Q and Volkow N. 2021. Increased risk of COVID-19 infection and mortality in people with mental disorders: Analysis from electronic health records in the United States. *World Psychiatry Online First* 2021: 1–7.

The World Bank Group. 2018. *Implementing the 2030 agenda. 2018 update*. The World Bank Group, Washington, DC.

World Health Organization. 2019. *WHO guideline recommendations on digital interventions for health system strengthening*. World Health Organization, Genève. License: CC BY-NC-SA 3.0 IGO.

World Health Organization. 2020a. www.who.int/en/.

World Health Organization. 2020b. *Coronavirus*. Geneva. www.who.int/health-topics/coronavirus.

World Health Organization. 2021. *COVID-19 and mandatory vaccination: Ethical considerations and caveats*. Policy Brief, Genève. 13 April 2021.

Yu P, Zhu J, Zhang Z et al. 2020. A familial cluster of infection associated with the 2019 novel coronavirus indicating possible person-to-person transmission during the incubation period. *The Journal of Infectious Diseases* 221 (11): 1757–1761.

8 Public Health as a Social Choice

The state of a population's health is deeply influenced by economic, social, political, and therefore, cultural factors. That is, social factors create and shape the patterns of health and disease. This principle of social epidemiology necessitates the adoption of clear public health measures, particularly in education, basic sanitation, infectious disease control, and social protection mechanisms, among others. If concerted, these effectors can have a decisive, positive impact on the quality of life, disease prevention, and life expectancy; that is, overall gains in health.

The principles underlying public health, which is the science and art of organizing communitarian health efforts, are in apparent contradiction with all forms of biological determinism, particularly genetic determinism. This has caused some tension between social epidemiology and techno sciences. This perspective seeks to improve the population's health conditions in a communitarian context. However, intuitively, the *real patient* always takes precedence over the *statistical patient* once the former is the ultimate object of public health and epidemiology than the latter, which is its operational instrument. Moreover, when we ethically reflect on the paradox of prevention, we can recognize that health policy and public health measures may or not bring substantial benefits to the individual patient. Some authors even advocate for the existence of a new ethic for public health, namely the importance of health promotion at crosscutting level throughout society as an ethical imperative of the health professions (Beauchamp and Steinbock 1999).

On a global scale, it is recognized today that globalization is not only an economic or cultural endeavour, but it is also an evolution of huge civilizational impact (Engebretsen and Heggen 2015). Environmental changes, water resources, biodiversity, or public health need coordinated strategies at the global level for the harmonious development of each human being.

Socioeconomic Status

Epidemiology refers to the study of distribution and determinants of health-related conditions in specific populations and their use for the control of health problems. From a sociological perspective, epidemiology in promoting public health is considered as a true instrument of social justice besides being an area of medicine (Coughlin and Beauchamp 1996). A priori, what is at stake is the recognition of

DOI: 10.4324/9781003241065-9

the importance of health sociology as a field of sociology that intends to deal with broad scope concepts such as the social role of the sick person, the experience of falling ill, the importance of medicalization (and quaternary prevention), and the various social constructions emerging from it, that is, the sociological study of health services at the organizational level. Possibly, both a reformulation of traditional health promotion strategies and a change of archetypes can happen, such as the concepts of risk factors, controlled clinical trials, or cost-benefit analyses. This is a different perspective of respect for social welfare that promotes responsibility with a view of solidarity. Thus, from this perspective, the old paradigm of health education policy, namely changing individual behavior, should be reassessed more as a consensual definition of the type of life that society intends and is worth living (Buchanan 2000).

As a clearly structured science, sociology rests on the concepts of social reproduction and social transformation. Indeed, the generations of people who constitute a particular society are a continuum because each generation slowly transforms itself due to several sociocultural factors.

Its methodological assumption, the *sociological imagination*, implies a rationale and detached analysis in due time that allows for the objective study of the evolution of humankind (Bird et al. 2000). Disease represents a unique milestone in each person's biography leading to a profound change in an individual's psychological state (Burlá et al. 2014). However, different people assume different roles in this context and in different diseases. These roles are categorized according to archetypes that are well defined by biomedicine and cause different alterations in the bio-psycho-social constitution of everyone. The English language recognizes this idiosyncrasy through these expressions: *disease*, *sickness*, and *illness*. The combination of signs and symptoms, that is, disease, becomes a sickness when the person perceives it as such and illness when the individual is recognized as socially incapacitated by the disease.

Cross-sector efforts may depend not only on the development of information infrastructure to monitor health inequalities but also on the implementation of clear and effective marketing strategies. Aggressive health education campaigns find ethical foundation in a higher social good that is to promote the health of citizens, inducing society to a radical change of conventional paradigms. But, in any case, and for whatever solution is adopted, the freedom of choice and consumption of adult persons should be respected provided they are fully informed of the harm caused by their choices. The implementation of a social policy with objectives of this nature goes beyond the competence of the government, thus requiring the active participation of the various associated social sectors. This is the assumption that only true cross-sector collaboration will permit achieving well-being, quality of life, and, therefore, health. It is important to keep in mind that the concept of health is not just the absence of disease itself but a holistic circumstance in which a person feels well, fit, able, and not limited by discomfort or disability.

The goals of health policy have not always been the same but, rather, change in response to economic, political, and social factors. Therefore, three major periods can be defined. In the second half of the 19th century when, in many developed countries, universal access to healthcare became a political objective, policy goals centered on structuring and organizing health units. Later, after World War II, the goals were essentially financial in nature and sought to increase the efficiency of the provision of health services (Williams 1994). Thus, the major objectives were minimizing health expenditures and controlling supplies through an efficient resource allocation policy (Harris 1998). Currently, in addition to these goals, health policy goals place special emphasis on the determination and control of risk factors and social determinants of health.

The considerable increase in average life expectancy in civilized societies is the paradigmatic example of this dynamic and evolutionary relationship between social factors and the health of a population. In essence, socioeconomic improvement, both individually and collectively, generates health benefits. Regardless of the overall quality of the health system, as perceived by citizens, there has been a notable increase in health indicators.

The relationship between the socioeconomic status of an individual and the emergence of health risk factors has long been clearly and unequivocally established. Even temporal evolution does not alter the essence of this reality, given that while the major causes of mortality have changed over the past few centuries, their association with socioeconomic status has remained constant. This situation manifests as early as the first years of the life of an individual. It is, according to Steven Gortmaker, the *first injustice* to be maintained and developed throughout life, even in old age. Thus, there is a life-long positive correlation between a person's socioeconomic status, average life expectancy, and other health indicators (Gortmaker and Wise 1997).

There are several ways in which a person of higher socioeconomic status can achieve greater health gains:

1   Better access to healthcare;
2   Higher quality treatment;
3   Better access to public health programs (e.g., vaccination and neoplasm screening);
4   Well-balanced, nutrient-rich diet (e.g., fruits and vegetables);
5   Fewer harmful practices (e.g., smoking and alcoholism);
6   Healthier overall lifestyle (e.g., physical exercise);
7   Housing in areas with high sanitization standards (e.g., drinking water and waste management);
8   High-quality primary and secondary education and consequent high level of general education and health literacy;
9   Higher levels of digital inclusion (World Health Organization 2019b).

Socioeconomic status, representing money, knowledge, prestige, and power, decreases the risk of morbidity and mortality. From the socioeconomic status perspective, the better-off adopt preventive and curative strategies to avoid disease risks, thereby mitigating the associated mortality. In this way, they can gradually improve their health and well-being. When discoveries emerge in the biomedical domain, such as measures to prevent cancer or cardiovascular disease, those who are socioeconomically better-off are more likely to adopt these discoveries primarily because they are more connected to digital society (European Union Agency for Fundamental Rights 2018). This is a reality in any society. In contrast, the worse-off tend to score lower in health promotion, even more when there are intersectional circumstances such as ethnicity or gender (Nunes 2020).

In more developed countries, the main causes of mortality have changed radically over the last two centuries. Cholera, tuberculosis, malaria, and other infectious diseases have given way to new epidemiological realities, namely the overwhelming growth of mortality due to cancer and cardiovascular disease. While centered on the human person as a social being, public health has progressively grown to recognize the constant dialogue between the human being and nature. It does not mean the recognition of intrinsic value to the environment; rather, it is to recognize that in its essence, human life is part of a whole and thus, inseparable from the commonwealth of life (Ledgerwood and Broadhurst 2000). With its many facets, the environment has earned the scrutiny and protection of society, particularly in the last decade. It is not only its contribution to health that is now being considered but also the inescapable fact that without a healthy and sustainable environment, human life is at stake. In a broad sense, the environment is, per se, everything that involves the human being in their interaction with society and nature (One Health). The United Nations has played a decisive role over the past few years through the establishment of the Sustainable Development Goals that put health and sustainable development at the epicenter of global policy decisions (United Nations 2020). This includes many aspects central to full human development such as the treatment of waste and toxic residues, basic sanitation, and the quality of drinking water (Capon and Corvalana 2018). In recent years, there has been a gradual improvement in the living conditions of the worldwide population. Therefore, a positive impact on health indicators on a global scale is expected (Adams 2016).

The implementation of a truly cross-sector policy requires the development of instruments to monitor health inequalities (GBD 2017 Mortality Collaborators 2018). The measurement of health status inequality within a population requires using appropriate indicators and empirical epidemiological evidence that focuses on their effective reduction. Social factors such as education, employment, income level, and housing are directly proportional to health indexes, in other words, ensuring that opportunities, orientations, skills, talents, and individual resources sustain and promote health, well-being, and quality of life. Moreover, the feeling of control over one's own life influences the state of health on a physical and mental level (Nunes et al. 2017).

In short, health is influenced by several factors: genetic, biological, behavioral, environmental, social, economic, and health services. In turn, these are determined by both individual and societal actions (Nunes and Rego 2014). However, the legal system of each nation-state can, and should, restrain the behavior of citizens either through punitive measures or through their pedagogical and therefore, preventive role. Only a concerted intervention in which all agents involved participate proactively may, in the future, lead to even better global health standards (Koplan et al. 2009).

Understanding the social determinants of health is essential for the transversal improvement of the health of any society and even more so, the global population. If there is no doubt that social factors create and shape the patterns of health and disease, then according to this paradigm, they do so predictably. Moreover, we can possibly say that this association has remained stable over time and regardless of the most prevalent type of disease, subsisted in cultures as diverse as the European, North American, or Eastern countries. Further, it persists even when risk factors such as alcohol, tobacco, obesity, or a sedentary lifestyle are excluded.

According to Wilkinson and Marmot (1998), the social determinants of health that complement certain biological and genetic factors include the following:

1   Economic and social gradients,
2   Ability to control the circumstances of life,
3   Start of healthy life and early development,
4   Existence of social and family support,
5   Existence of stable employment,
6   Absence of addictions,
7   Consumption of nutrient-rich food and other healthy products, and
8   Use of healthy means of transportation.

There is a significant association between an individual's socioeconomic status and the health of their spouse and children, mortality in the retirement age, and accidental mortality. Parents with higher levels of education provide their children with greater academic success, which indirectly influences health. Experimental evidence supports the association between social class and the rate of mortality, morbidity, and disability (GBD 2017 SDG Collaborators 2018). This relationship finds its foundation in the effect of socioeconomic status on health (social causation); even though there is an inverse relationship, the effect of health on social status (social selection) is also important. This vicious circle of health→well-being-success is based, in essence, on three fundamental components:

1   Education,
2   Employment/occupation (advanced capabilities), and
3   Income level.

Education includes years of schooling and academic achievement throughout primary, secondary, and higher education. Yet, it also has its roots in the example set by parents and other social symbols that become decisive in the structuring of one's personality. A high level of education indicates knowledge, capacity, and the apprehension of values and norms of behavior which enable both acquiring basic health information and obtaining critical credentials for obtaining employment;

hence, including education is important for responsible citizenship in primary education (Nunes et al. 2015).

Variables such as the level of education, the quality of basic education, and the existence of effective health education programs (including nutritional education, sex education, education for the prevention of drug, tobacco, and alcohol abuse) are part of this dynamic by decisively contributing to the sustained improvement of the health of a population. The educational level of a population, expressed as a proportion of individuals between the ages of 15 and 64 who completed at least compulsory schooling, has been improving globally. However, along with this global improvement in the level of education, the high rate of illiteracy must be mentioned; some studies suggest that only 84% of the population can read and write (Bulc et al. 2019).

From the health promotion perspective, the daily occupation of each person is important. Different work categories, namely total and partial employment as well as professional prestige or hierarchical position within an organization, are decisive factors. Further, the importance of unemployment should not be overlooked, or the inability to work due to physical or mental incapacity, retirement age, or domestic obligations. Other activities, in addition or as an alternative to formal employment, such as domestic activities or leisure activities for elderly and retired persons, or social solidarity activities are important factors in promoting health. Moreover, with the advent of the digital economy, robotics, and the introduction of artificial intelligence, and quantum computing in production processes (Boman and Kruse 2017), it is estimated that the employment problem is one of the great challenges of this new millennium since a large portion of traditional jobs are rapidly being replaced. Therefore, the relationship between socioeconomic status and employment needs a new approach on a global scale (Independent High-Level Expert Group on Artificial Intelligence 2019).

Undoubtedly, the level of economic income, even in the medium term, can condition these variables qualitatively and quantitatively. These are factors such as salary or other income, productive activity, and material possessions. The concept of social inequality is also relevant in this matter. A study by Richard Wilkinson (1992) has shown that average life expectancy at birth is considerably lower in countries that provide a substantially lower share of income to 70% of the population (who are in worse socioeconomic conditions). When most of the income goes to 30% of the population and is not evenly distributed, the average life expectancy of the entire population is considerably compromised. Thus, life span extension is indexed to the income gap of a given population. However, modern societies should not disregard the *emotional salary*, that is, all those noneconomic rewards that contribute decisively for self-actualization at work. This is the reason why advanced capabilities should be promoted at work.

The distinction between health and satisfaction, that is, degree of contentment with the current situation, is also useful. Although overlapping concepts, one can be satisfied with the circumstances of life even if they do not correspond to a true state of physical, psychological, or social well-being. Moreover, physical and mental health should be considered as two sides of an indivisible whole because:

1   Conditions that protect physical health (e.g., education) also protect mental health;
2   Each of these varieties decisively influences the other, for example, chronic diseases cause depression, and in turn, depression leads to the lack of physical exercise, poor diet, and health risks;
3   Symptoms such as tiredness, shortness of breath, and palpitations may result from both physical and psychological illness;
4   The nervous and the endocrine systems bridge the gap between our physical and mental dimensions;
5   Direct social disadvantage, concerning education, housing, diet, access to healthcare, etc.; and
6   The social condition is intrinsically disturbing, and hence, its influence on the organism, especially the nervous and immune systems.

The concept of relative deprivation refers to this purpose. The lower a person is in the socioeconomic gradient, the more demotivation and subjective sense of marginalization this person feels. This feeling is related to one's relative position in society, although it may or may not be based on fact. What is at stake is the possibility of physiological and therefore, pathological consequences arising from a lack of control over one's life. The hierarchical position of an individual in society, per se, is a source of stress. Once subjected to this institutional hierarchy, anyone can become vulnerable to a diverse set of circumstances, resulting in multiple negative states from physical, psychological, and emotional perspectives.

Income inequality, and hence socioeconomic status, is a more important factor in the average life expectancy of the population than the average level of per capita income (United Nations 2019). Relative position in society prevails over absolute income likely due to the psycho-affective effect of social position and hierarchical dependence. From a sociological perspective, stratification is a more important social determinant of health than employment, income, or even the prestige of a citizen. Further, in all societies there are huge income disparities between men and women (World Economic Forum 2019). Gender-sensitive policies in all aspects of public policy are therefore of fundamental importance for an effective promotion of health (UNESCO 2014).

Another association of the greatest importance in health, besides inequalities (namely the income and gender gap), is the existence of a social support network; this is reflected, among other things, in the population's average life expectancy. Social support of persons in need protects them against health risks and promotes prevention strategies. The family's role, as the nuclear unit of society, has received attention from social epidemiology for being a decisive factor in the protection of health. The family contributes to the education of any person in a decisive and integral way. Its appreciation is instrumental in promoting social cohesion and the sustained improvement of a society's health indicators, regardless of the specific concept of family and the cultural reality in which it is inserted. Therefore, protecting families from poverty is of fundamental importance. Notwithstanding the fact that poverty is multidimensional, techniques such as the Alkire–Foster method should be implemented to address this issue (Alkire and Foster 2011). Further, child-specific deprivation, namely monetary child poverty and material deprivation, should be considered as essential elements for truly promoting health (Chzhen et al. 2016).

Implementing measures to reduce social inequalities and improve the average level of socioeconomic status is not the sole responsibility of the family; the family must also contribute to increasing literacy levels of the children. Moreover, a detailed assessment and interpretation of data on this subject appear to show a marked improvement in the household's role at the global scale, though there is still no concerted cross-sector intervention targeting this issue (Oni et al. 2019). The implementation of a policy that is sensitive to the social determinants of health should make a decisive contribution to the quality of life in various countries (European Parliament 2011).

Social Determinants of Health

The differences in health in the different countries of the world result, on the one hand, from differences in individual behavior and, on the other hand, from social inequalities (Secretary's Advisory Committee 2010).

The major determinants of health in developed countries are related to the excessive consumption of tobacco and alcohol, high cholesterol levels, and obesity rates. Epidemiologists agree that the most influential factor in the health status of an individual is lifestyle; therefore, it is essential to define and implement measures to promote health and protection from disease. In this context, programs focusing on the prevention of tobacco and alcohol consumption and the promotion of healthy eating have been already developed in most countries.

Nutrition as a determinant of health stems from the ability of healthy eating to prevent major causes of mortality and morbidity, particularly cardiovascular and neoplastic diseases. The development of health protection programs aimed at improving the quality of nutrition is a core element for improving the survival of a population and for improving the quality of life of the citizens in developed societies. The efforts made are mainly due to the awareness that the burden of the disease associated with poor nutrition is significant today. In the past decades, there has been a decrease in the levels of premature mortality. While this was influenced by a change in dietary habits, there is still a wide range of preventive strategies remaining at this level, namely primary healthcare.

For example, some epidemiological studies have shown that despite the efforts made to date, one-third of people living in Europe are overweight. Further, depending on the country, there has been an increase of 10% to 40% in the number of overweight individuals over the past decades. Numerous international projects have been developed toward formulating guidelines for the implementation of dietary norms, that is, projects to develop nutrition strategies that have an impact on public health and carry out an evaluation of the policies previously defined. The aim is to improve the nutritional status of populations in specific societies. In addition, on a global scale, similar programs must be implemented to positively change citizens' lifestyles (Cole and Fielding 2007). The guidelines for action fall on the continuing training of primary and secondary school teachers to encourage students to adopt more active and healthy lifestyles and in the nutrition education of the population. This strategy serves a double purpose. On the one hand, promoting a healthy diet regarding the excessive consumption of saturated fats, salt, sugar, and alcohol and on the other hand, decreasing the incidence of obesity in the population.

In the context of assessing the impact of dietary habits on individual and collective health, the importance of alcohol consumption in many countries warrants consideration. A study on the global burden of disease sponsored by the World Health Organization (WHO) and the World Bank found that "alcohol-related death and disability are responsible for high costs to life and longevity." Besides causing numerous chronic diseases at the physical and psychological level, excessive consumption of alcohol has economic and social consequences for the individual and society. The most common effects are related to the performance of family activities, work, and public order phenomena.

Some studies aim to determine the social effects of the increase in consumption of one liter of alcohol per capita and find that:

1   Accident mortality rates are influenced by alcohol consumption, with a statistically significant positive association between these two variables.
2   There is the same kind of relationship between alcohol and homicide rates, and gender violence.
3   As it is now clearly demonstrated, alcohol in small quantities can have beneficial effects on health, especially concerning the prevention of cardiovascular disease.

Within the context of the relative failure of preventive and pedagogical measures, it is necessary to adopt measures that reduce alcohol consumption and the problems related to its consumption. If implemented, in the short term, these initiatives can lead to a reduction of workplace and traffic accidents, hospital emergency admissions (from excessive consumption and associated accidents), and general hospital admissions. The target populations of such campaigns are young people, pregnant or breastfeeding women, and individuals with mental disorders.

Indeed, the guidelines should refer to the need to:

1   Develop campaigns in each country about alcohol consumption;
2   Develop regional networks for community prevention and evaluation of alcohol problem;

3   Review the legislation on the advertising and sale of alcoholic beverages to minors;
4   Improve the training of professionals from different sectors of society; and
5   Increase and value attitudes that aim to prevent traffic and work accidents, and prevent gender violence.

Further, the regular consumption of alcohol during childhood, even in small quantities, can affect the child's brain which continues developing into their early twenties (Department of Health 2019). Moreover, alcohol can dramatically affect the performance at school. Perhaps, for this reason, some epidemiologists consider that alcohol represents a major public health problem related to addictions (Department of Health and Human Services 2019).

Smoking is also a major cause of mortality and morbidity in many countries. According to the WHO, tobacco kills more than 8 million people each year (World Health Organization 2019a). More than 7 million of those deaths are the result of direct tobacco use while around 1.2 million are the result of nonsmokers being exposed to second-hand smoke. It is estimated that approximately 15% of cancers in developed countries are related to tobacco consumption (Cancer Research UK 2019). Recent data indicate a decrease in the percentage of smokers worldwide. Indeed, the global prevalence of tobacco smoking among people aged ≥ 15 years reveals a prevalence of 26.9% in 2000 and a prevalence of 18.7% in 2020 (World Health Organization 2018a). However, around 80% of the world's 1.1 billion smokers live in low- and middle-income countries. Efforts to combat smoking at the global level conform to two types of preventive strategies: a) information/disclosure and b) legislation. Smoking prevention is crucial for the reduction of cancer, and therefore, different programs have devoted a part of their activity to interventions in this field over the past few years (European Observatory on Health Systems and Policies 2006).

At the legislative level, directives have been established that require labeling tobacco products with health warnings and/or indications of tar and nicotine levels along with other measures such as forbidding to smoke in public areas. Further, legislations that increase tobacco taxes and advertising restrictions aimed toward discouraging tobacco consumption, particularly among adolescents, have been introduced. The efficacy of these information and legislation-based efforts should manifest as:

1   Decrease in smoking behavior in the general population, particularly in young people;
2   Increase of former smokers; and
3   Protection of nonsmokers from exposure to second-hand smoke.

In this context, the main targets for 2025 should be to increase the prevalence of nonsmoking young people and former smokers by 10% and 2.5%, respectively.

Likewise, additional efforts should be made to establish policies that raise aware-ness among teachers and healthcare professionals about their pedagogical role; this will indirectly contribute to increase the prevalence of former smokers. Among other operational practices, the goal should be to:

1   Increase citizens' awareness of the harmful effects of tobacco and raise public awareness;
2   Encourage the establishment of tobacco-free health and education facilities;
3   Promote international scientific meetings about smoking;
4   Preventing tobacco use in schools and workplaces;
5   Strengthen legislative measures; and
6   Mobilize professional associations through the decisive role of the physician.

Drug addiction is another public health issue of great concern. The use of illicit drugs has been the target of numerous preventive policies aimed toward reduc-ing the impact of their excessive use, both physically and mentally. These poli-cies have been developed to be sustainable and include programs of action at the international level. Many countries attempted to fight drug abuse by setting clear policies for prevention, treatment, and social reintegration. It is necessary to define strategic lines of action with the purpose of reducing the consumption of illicit drugs. Thus, the main objectives are:

1   The need to reverse or at least reduce the growing trend in drug demand;
2   Increase the proportion of young people who never or only sporadically used illicit substances;
3   Ensure access to substitution programs for all heroin addicts with therapeutic indications;
4   Ensure access to the network of specialized care for all drug addicts who seek treatment; and
5   Strengthen harm reduction measures to prevent the spread of infectious dis-eases and bring drug addicts closer to healthcare structures.

Toward this end, some countries have implemented facilities with specialized pro-fessional support (physicians, nurses, and psychosocial professionals) to minimize the impact of illicit drugs on the health of the drug addict and the transmission of vectors associated with infectious diseases (Belackova and Salmon 2017). How-ever, the implementation of these drug consumption rooms (i.e., supervised injec-tion centers) has generated some concern for two reasons: First, it is now proven that a policy to reduce illicit drug use rests essentially on preventive strategies during childhood and adolescence. Second, it is because of the symbolic, negative value of its implementation; according to this line of thinking, by adopting this strategy, the message society conveys to citizens is that the use of illicit drugs is not intrinsically negative and, to a certain extent, should even be favored, given the right to self-determination.

However, for a few decades, in Europe and elsewhere, there have been drug consumption rooms where illicit drugs can be used under the supervision of trained personnel (Belackova et al. 2018). The central objective is to:

1   Reduce the acute risks of disease transmission due to unhygienic injection practices;
2   Prevent deaths from drug overdose; and
3   Bring together high-risk consumers and drug treatment services as well as other health and social services.

Importantly, the impact of these measures should be carefully monitored to ensure that they are achieving their intended objectives (Skolnik 2015). Within the scope of policies for the prevention and reduction of risks and minimization of damage, programs for controlled consumption aim to increase asepsis in intravenous consumption and consequently reduce the inherent risks of this form of consumption, as well as the promotion of proximity to consumers. From a public policy perspective, the consumer is not considered as a criminal, but as someone who needs helps from society and the health system. Trafficking only should be a crime. Despite successive efforts, indications of drug use, associated mortality, and prevalence of the human immunodeficiency virus (HIV) are still the subject of intense concern; further, different countries have different results in this field. Regarding AIDS, new HIV infections have been reduced by 40% since the peak in 1997. Since 2010, new HIV infections have declined by an estimated 16%, from 2.1 million to 1.7 million in 2018 (UNAIDS 2019).

Within this framework, the defined goals can be grouped into six broad categories:

1   Primary prevention;
2   Reduction of risks, public health, and consumer health;
3   Treatment;
4   Social reintegration;
5   Statistical and epidemiological research and information; and
6   International cooperation.

Social inequality and stratification, prosperity, and socioeconomic status are interdependent variables that determine the living conditions of each citizen. Therefore, both the conditions and the environment in which each person lives and works are core elements for the harmonious development of personality and the protection of health (World Health Organization 2018b). Factors such as the type of housing and its existence, the number of residents, the presence of drinking water and basic sanitation, the presence of fresh air, and the reduction of exposure to environmental and workplace toxins have been, for a long time, the subject of study in the fields of epidemiology and social epidemiology. What is in question, among other measures, is the control of vectors of infectious diseases, the promotion of a healthy working environment, or the implementation of measures that protect biodiversity, and thus, the improvement of the quality of life of citizens.

Overpopulated housing, for example, usually causes great physical disruption, and thus, translates into health problems for the individual, the family, and the community. The reverse should also be considered: being sick, bedridden, or incapacitated, or having an acute or chronic illness requires decent housing conditions that allow for emotional well-being and thus, help the sick persons overcome their situation. The association between poor living conditions and poverty, and psychoaffective disorders, such as depression and anxiety, is well established (Lund et al. 2010). Poor living conditions, poor housing, and lack of heating are good examples as they facilitate both the development of respiratory diseases and the appearance of addictive behaviors such as alcoholism and drug addiction. The type of housing is another factor that clearly and unequivocally denotes that social inequality separates people into groups that are associated with different health risks and different social rewards. Over the past few years, there has been a substantial improvement on a global scale in the promotion of a housing policy that discriminates positively (i.e., reverse discrimination) and as such caters to the worst-off in society. Indeed, the rapid urbanization of many countries is a landmark of the economic globalization and a symptom of the growing middle class worldwide (Zhang 2016).

Conclusion

Socioeconomic status is a decisive factor in human development. Primarily, there is a direct correlation between this status and levels of health education. In fact, health literacy assumes relevance in contemporary society for diverse reasons. First, because full and responsible citizenship can only be achieved when citizens have a level of education and training that allows them to have a fruitful and self-realized life. Education, culture, and knowledge are, of course, essential tools for including everyone regardless of social and family conditions. Equal opportunities can be only achieved if there are high levels of literacy and civic culture (Sen 1999). Despite specific contingencies, most societies have made huge strides in the last decades by universalizing access to basic and secondary education and by promoting the conditions necessary for young people to opt for higher education.

Meanwhile, the sociodemographic structure of civilized societies is undergoing a profound transformation, with a marked fall in birth rates and a progressively aging population associated with a consistent increase in average life expectancy. The combination of these factors, that is, the relative decrease of informal caregivers, namely the family, and increased longevity, calls for well-defined social policies for active aging with genuine involvement of different social actors, such as government, academia, institutions of the third sector (social economy), and social entrepreneurs.

However, health literacy is also an individual responsibility. Indeed, the development of better living conditions over the past few years also means that the senior population anticipates some of the predictable health problems of old age, preparing for the lifestyle that best meets their needs and aspirations. This ethic of responsibility, both individual and collective, requires innovative forms of health education so that the impact of aging and associated conditions (e.g., increased prevalence of dementia) are optimized to provide a happy and harmonic life in old age. This global, public health-oriented perspective is fundamental for the construction of modern, prosperous, and developed societies.

References

Adams V. 2016. *Metrics: What counts in global health.* Duke University Press, Durham.

Alkire S and Foster J. 2011. Counting and multidimensional poverty measurement. *Journal of Public Economics* 95 (7): 476–487.

Beauchamp D and Steinbock B. 1999. *New Ethics for the public's health.* Oxford University Press, New York.

Belackova V and Salmon AM. 2017. Overview of international literature – supervised injecting centers & drug consumption rooms – Issue 1. Uniting Medically Supervised Injecting Center, Sydney.

Belackova V, Salmon AM, Schatz E et al. 2018. Online census of drug consumption rooms (DCRs) as a setting to address HCV: Current practice and future capacity. International Network of Drug Consumption Rooms, Correlation Network/Uniting Medically Supervised Injecting Centre, Amsterdam.

Bird C, Conrad P and Fremont A. 2000. *Handbook of medical sociology.* Prentice-Hall, New Jersey, 5th edition.

Boman M and Kruse E. 2017. Supporting global health goals with information and communications technology. *Global Health Action* 10 (3): 6–13.

Buchanan D. 2000. *An ethic for health promotion. Rethinking the sources of human well-being.* Oxford University Press, New York.

Bulc B, Al-Wahdani B, Bustreo F et al. 2019. Urgency for transformation: Youth engagement in global health. *The Lancet* 7: 1–2.

Burlá C, Rego G and Nunes R. 2014. Alzheimer, dementia and the living will: A proposal. Medicine, *Healthcare and Philosophy* 17 (3): 389–395.

Cancer Research UK. 2019. Tobacco statistics. www.cancerresearchuk.org/health-profes sional/cancer-statistics/risk/tobacco [Accessed 10 July 2019].

Capon A and Corvalana C. 2018. Climate change and health: Global issue, local responses. *Public Health Research & Practice* 28 (4): 1–3.

Chzhen Y, de Neubourg C, Plavgo I et al. 2016. Child poverty in the European Union: The multiple overlapping deprivation analysis approach (EU-MODA). *Child Indicators Research* 9: 335–356. https://doi.org/10.1007/s12187-015-9321-7.

Cole BL and Fielding JE. 2007. Health impact assessment: A tool to help policy makers understand health beyond health care. *Annual Review of Public Health* 28: 393–412.

Coughlin S and Beauchamp T. 1996. *Ethics and epidemiology.* Oxford University Press, New York.

Department of Health. 2019. Alcohol and the developing brain. Government of Western Australia. https://healthywa.wa.gov.au/Articles/F_I/Information-for-parents-alcohol-and-the-developing-brain. [Accessed 09 August 2019].

Department of Health and Human Services. 2019. HHS action plan to reduce racial and ethnic health disparities. A nation free of disparities in health and health care. http://minorityhealth.hhs.gov/npa.

Engebretsen E and Heggen K. 2015. Powerful concepts in global health. Comment on "Knowledge, moral claims and the exercise of power in global health." *International Journal of Health Policy and Management* 4 (2): 115–117.

European Observatory on Health Systems and Policies. 2006. Health in all policies: Prospects and potentials. www.euro.who.int/__data/assets/pdf_file/0003/109146/E89260.pdf [PDF – 1.23 MB].

European Parliament. 2011. Directive 2011/24/EU of the European parliament and of the council of 9 March 2011 on the application of patients' rights in cross-border healthcare. https://eur-lex.europa.eu/legal-content/EN/TXT/?uri=CELEX%3A32011L0024.

European Union Agency for Fundamental Rights. 2018. BigData: Discrimination in data-supported decision making. http://fra.europa.eu/en/publication/2018/big-data-discrimination.

GBD 2017 Mortality Collaborators. 2018. Global, regional, and national age-sex-specific mortality and life expectancy, 1950–2017: A systematic analysis for the global burden of disease study 2017. *The Lancet* 392: 1684–1735.

GBD 2017 SDG Collaborators. 2018. Measuring progress from 1990 to 2017 and projecting attainment to 2030 of the health-related sustainable development goals for 195 countries and territories: A systematic analysis for the global burden of disease study 2017. *The Lancet* 392: 2091–2138.

Gortmaker S and Wise P. 1997. The first injustice: Socioeconomic disparities, health services technology, and infant mortality. *Annual Review of Sociology* 23: 147–170.

Harris J. 1998. *Micro-allocation: Deciding between patients. A companion to bioethics, blackwell companions to philosophy*, Helga Kuhse and Peter Singer (Editors). Blackwell Publishers, Oxford.

Independent High-Level Expert Group on Artificial Intelligence set up by the European Commission. 2019. Ethics guidelines for trustworthy AI. European Commission, Brussels. Document made public on April 8, 2019.

Koplan JP, Bond TC, Merson MH et al. 2009. Towards a common definition of global health. *The Lancet* 373 (9679): 1993–1995.

Ledgerwood G and Broadhurst A. 2000. *Environment, ethics and the corporation*. Macmillan Press Ltd, London.

Lund C, Breen A, Flisher A et al. 2010. Poverty and common mental disorders in low and middle income countries: A systematic review. *Social Science & Medicine* 71 (3): 517–528.

Nunes R. 2020. Addressing gender inequality to promote basic human rights and development: A global perspective, *CEDIS Working Papers* 2020 (1). http://cedis.fd.unl.pt/blog/project/addressing-gender-inequality-to-promote-basic-human-rights-and-development-a-global-perspective/.

Nunes R, Duarte I, Santos C et al. 2015. Education for values and bioethics. *SpringerPlus*. DOI: 10.1186/s40064-015-0815-z.

Nunes R, Nunes SB and Rego G. 2017. Healthcare as a universal right. *Journal of Public Health* 25: 1–9.

Nunes R and Rego G. 2014. Priority setting in health care: A complementary approach. *Health Care Analysis* 22: 292–303.

Oni T, Yudkin J, Fonn S et al. 2019. Global public health starts at home: Upstream approaches to global health training. *The Lancet* 7: 301–302.

Secretary's Advisory Committee on Health Promotion and Disease Prevention Objectives for 2020. 2010. Healthy people 2020: An opportunity to address the societal determinants of health in the United States. www.healthypeople.gov/2010/hp2020/advisory/ SocietalDeterminantsHealth.htm.

Sen A. 1999. *Development as freedom.* Knopf, New York.

Skolnik R. 2015. *Global health 101. Essential public health series.* Jones & Bartlett Learning, Burlington, 3rd edition.

UNAIDS. 2019. Global HIV & AIDS statistics – 2019 fact sheet. www.unaids.org/en/ resources/fact-sheet [Accessed 9 September 2019].

UNESCO. 2014. *UNESCO priority gender equality action plan 2014–2021.* UNESCO, Paris.

United Nations. 2019. *Human development report 2019. Beyond income, beyond averages, beyond today: Inequalities in human development in the 21st century.* United Nations Development Programme, New York.

United Nations. 2020. Sustainable development goals. www.un.org/sustainabledevelop ment/sustainable-development-goals/ [Accessed 12 January 2021].

Wilkinson R. 1992. Income distribution and life expectancy. *British Medical Journal* 304: 165–168.

Wilkinson R and Marmot M. 1998. *Social determinants of health: The solid facts.* World Health Organization, New York.

Williams A. 1994. *Economics, society, and health care ethics. Principles of health care ethics,* Raanan Gillon (Editor). John Wiley & Sons Ltd, London.

World Economic Forum. 2019. *Global gender gap report 2020.* World Economic Forum, Geneva.

World Health Organization. 2018a. WHO global report on trends in prevalence of tobacco smoking 2000–2025. World Health Organization, Genève, 2nd edition.

World Health Organization. 2018b. *WHO housing and health guidelines.* World Health Organization, Genève.

World Health Organization. 2019a. Tobacco: Key facts. www.who.int/news-room/fact-sheets/detail/tobacco [Accessed 9 September 2019].

World Health Organization. 2019b. *WHO guideline recommendations on digital interventions for health system strengthening.* World Health Organization, Genève. License: CC BY-NC-SA 3.0 IGO.

Zhang XQ. 2016. The trends, promises and challenges of urbanisation in the world. *Habitat International* 54 (3): 241–252.

9 New Public Management in Healthcare

In modern countries, healthcare is usually considered a social right. Different systems of healthcare delivery have been implemented in accordance with this perspective. Equity in access has been the paradigm of healthcare systems in most liberal democracies. Equity means that the principle of justice involved in the distribution of health is primarily based on personal need. The pursuit of equity usually implies a reduction in unjust disparities between individual citizens or social groups (Daniels and Sabin 2002).

Nevertheless, the increasing costs of healthcare, mainly due to scientific and technological developments, medical malpractice, the increasing age of the population, and consumerism, make the establishment of priorities an economic and even social imperative (Mullen and Spurgeon 2000). In this vein, the steady debate between equity and efficiency led to the introduction of the rules and principles of new public management in the provision of healthcare. However, the search for efficiency has also led to the rise of healthcare regulations in most developed countries to monitor and enforce rules and guidelines.

Government Failures and Public Choice

Even before World War II, most developed countries relied on their governments (on the various levels of public administration) to satisfy certain essential goods that traditionally were not at the mercy of the market forces. These were namely, services particularly valued by the population, such as health, education, social security, and environmental protection, among many others. Therefore, there is an equation that combines public services with the public sector and the public spending in accordance with a particular view of a public service ethos. This ethical/social background relies on the following acknowledged governance principles (Davis 1998):

1 A fair and reasonably egalitarian distribution of income,
2 Equality of access to services,
3 Discrimination in favor of meritorious activity,
4 Non-profit-oriented decision-making,

DOI: 10.4324/9781003241065-10

5   Dealings with costumers based on the customer's interest, not the commercial interest of the supplier,
6   Stakeholder type personnel policies,
7   Non-payment of profit, [and]
8   Co-operative industry relationships.

However, this equation has been challenged by many scholars, politicians, and other social agents, especially in the last quarter of the 20th century; these actors suggest that the traditional paradigm that the government acts *in the public interest* is incorrect, considering growing government failures. It is important to point out the main arguments behind those criticisms, considering that some are the most influential theories and scholars in the subject, and to try to determine if these arguments are convincing and to identify the main solutions proposed to guarantee the public interest.

The main criticisms of the traditional government model are related to several key issues. First, the existence of government failures in the provision of essential goods such as health, education, justice, and social services questions the public providers' capacity to respond effectively to citizens' preferences. It is presumed that responsiveness should be regarded as a key element of a new ideological platform of public policy, which is necessary for political decisions to be in substantial harmony with citizens' wishes. Indeed, government failures are particularly difficult to accept in liberal democracies because of society's high demand index and the systematic scrutiny of the media. This lack of responsiveness may be related not only to the shortage of services and huge waiting lists but also to issues such as bureaucracy and unfriendliness (Le Grand 2007). However, and unsurprisingly, there is a generalized crisis of public trust in developed societies directed even at our most familiar institutions and office holders (O'Neill 2006), even if the process of social choice is a complex one (Arrow 1963a; Bossert and Weymark 2004).

Second, and equally as important as the first issue, is the lack of sustainability of several public services due to many factors, such as inefficient resource allocation policies (allocative inefficiency). This inefficient use of public resources (gathered through taxation) is associated both with complex structure of public services administration and with the self-interest of politicians and of some public officials that frequently regard the public interest as a second choice.

There are also civilizational factors that have contributed to this evolution in many countries. For example, growing life expectancy is a dramatic driver of the increase in public spending in healthcare and social security. This driver is expected to further pressure the complex social systems of modern countries as life expectancy continues to increase in the next decades.

However, the traditional view of the government mainly anchored in a bureaucratic model of organizations was a major organizational achievement. Conceptually, the theory of bureaucracy (Max Weber, 1864–1920) is one of the main pillars of the traditional model of public administration that is historically related to the provision of public services. Essentially, this model is characterized by the subordination of public officials to elected political leaders, where the staff of an organization is constituted by workers recruited primarily for their technical pro-file and expertise in accordance with true public interest. This theory holds:

1   The division of labor, considering functional specialization;
2   The well-defined hierarchy of authority;
3   The existence of rules that precisely define the rights and duties of each worker and procedures that resolve the situations that arise at work;
4   That relationships at work should be impersonal to avoid emotional factors from affecting the quality of decisions;
5   Admissions and promotions should be decided considering the technical competence of the candidates and not, for example, family relations, friendship, or personal charisma.

Indeed, bureaucracy theory intends to achieve the highest possible efficiency of any public organization. For instance, Max Weber holds that

> The decisive reason for the advance of the bureaucratic organization has always been its purely technical superiority over any other form of organization. The fully developed bureaucratic mechanism compares with other organizations exactly as does the machine with non-mechanical modes of production. Precision, speed, unambiguity, knowledge of the files, continuity, discretion, unity, strict subordination, reduction of friction and personal costs – these are raised to the optimum point in the strictly bureaucratic organization
>
> Hughes 1998

Proponents claimed that the fully developed bureaucratic mechanism is always technically superior to other forms of organization through a clear, top-down chain of command and control. In addition, the division of labor is based on rules and well-defined assumptions, such as functional specialization and impersonality in industrial relations. However, even if it can allow overcoming the characteristic problems of other types of organizations (e.g., family influence and no appreciation of merit), the coordination of activities, in many cases, failed to generate adequate productive efficiency levels. This was partly due to the excessive size and hierarchy of the activities, its monopolistic structure, and the absence of valid performance indicators (Niskanen 1994). Indeed, not forgetting the importance of this perspective in developed societies, the multiplicity and complexity of many public services that have emerged in all countries in the past decades have ultimately resulted in huge organizational inefficiency.

The bureaucratic mechanism has also been challenged due to the lack of political accountability, public accountability, responsiveness to society, and empowerment of the people and because it does not promote a clear separation between politics and public administration (Nunes et al. 2011). One of the reasons why public administration is considered inefficient is the fact that bureaucrats are often motivated by their own interests and not by the citizens' interests. Other reasons are related to the excessive dimension of some public agencies, besides the lack of performance indicators of the developed activities, where the chain of command between the elected politician and public official reverses, demanding more resources than those expected for the development of that activity. In public healthcare systems, for instance, its large dimension brings about another perspective of inefficiency, that is, the duplication of services or even their underutilization due to a lack of strategic planning in the conception and distribution of healthcare facilities.

Even so, there are important reasons to consider the necessity of an adequate public sector to deliver high-quality public services and that these services should be financed mainly by taxation and not by charging the consumer directly. In accordance with Davis (1998), "the impossibility of charging for everything," "the problem of price discrimination," and even "the failure of private capital markets" justifies this approach. Indeed, and beyond considerations of the ideological and redistributive nature of universal access to certain economic goods, the financing of many activities valued by most people is sometimes more feasible if done through taxes than if implemented using the logic of the user/payer. Eventually, it is carried out according to the criteria of justice since taxes are more than proportional (progressive) in relation to the income of individual citizens. Redistribution through taxes makes access to public services fairer and more equitable.

Given these developments, competing visions on how to reform the public sector consistently and voluntarily, ensure access to high-quality public services, and guarantee efficiency in public spending and its value-for-money began to emerge gradually. The public choice theory is one of the main contributions in this field. As suggested by the Nobel Laureate in Economics James M. Buchanan, this theory, as a domain that is midway between economics and political science, in fact refers to a theory of governmental failure: the government, or broadly, the political organization, fails to satisfy the ideal criteria of efficiency and equity (Buchanan and Tullock 1962). Indeed and as stated by Gordon Tullock (2005):

> The view that the individual bureaucrat is not attempting to maximize the public interest very vigorously but is attempting to maximize his own utility just as vigorously as you and I, have been held for a very long time by most people in the backs of their minds. But bringing it into formal theory is a public choice accomplishment.

According to Mueller (2008), "Public Choice has been defined as the application of the methodology of economics to the study of politics. This definition suggests that public choice is an inherently interdisciplinary field, and so it is." In contrast, Hill (1999) states that "Public choice is best defined as the application of the rational choice model to non-market decision-making."

The problem is not only the lack of efficiency per se but also that the growing inefficiency levels lead to overall unsustainability of the state, namely the accomplishment of its social obligations. Governmental failure is at the level of public service delivery (social functions and sovereignty responsibilities); however, it is also a failure to be the main driver of economic competition and global development because of being overweighed by public spending (Congleton 2004).

To address this problem, several solutions have been proposed, namely the introduction of new public management transversely across the public administration. New public management is more than just another reform of public administration. According to its proponents, it is not only a deep internal transformation of the public sector but also a conceptual approach to overcome some of the major problems in the interface between society and the government. New public management relies on the creation of an internal market (quasi-market). According to Julian Le Grand (2007):

> A quasi-market is like a market in the sense that there are independent providers competing for custom within it. But it differs from a normal market in at least one keyway. This is that users do not come to a quasi-market with their own resources to purchase goods and services, as with a normal market. Instead, the services are paid for by the state, but with the money following users' choices through the form of a voucher, an earmarked budget or a funding formula.

Meanwhile, the purchasing and provision of goods are split, private and public firms compete for output-based contracts (instead of input-based financing of public agencies alone), and innovation in the governance arrangements of public organizations is seen as an important aspect of reform. Thus, more autonomy is granted to managers and institutions, namely an *earned autonomy* (Lipsey 2005). Incentive payments, corporatization of public services, and even public/private partnerships (medium- to long-term ventures, where risk is shared, and responsibilities are clearly determined) were proposed as innovative measures.

One of the key features of new public management is the introduction of competition (and even choice) between different agents. However, this perspective may challenge some of the presuppositions of the public services equation suggested by Evan Davis. In particular, it is the equality of access to services, discrimination in favor of meritorious activity, nonprofit-oriented decision-making, avoiding the commercial interest of the supplier, a stakeholder approach to personnel policies, and the nonpayment of profit and a cooperative industry relationship. That is, competition should not be regarded as an end. The introduction of competitive market rules must be seen as a tool to generate competitiveness and ensure the economic sustainability of the system regarding the efficient use of taxes. Moreover, it should concern competition for the market (public financing) and not the competition within a market in the traditional sense. Further, government contracts must be strictly regulated (Cullis and Jones 2009).

However, there is still some dispute regarding how much choice consumers should have. As suggested by David Lipsey (2005), "choice and efficiency in public services may conflict" as, sometimes, there must be over-provision of public services, and therefore the true question might be "are the extra efficiencies you get from competition and choice greater than the inefficiencies required by having plenty of slack in the system?"

In summary, one question is fundamental. How do we ensure the nuclear and irreducible functions of the state? How do we adapt the welfare state to effectively protect valuable community assets, such as health or education? Or, how do we ensure that the transformation of a provider state model evolves into a regulatory state model (Majone 1994, 1997) to overcome known problems of competition and choice, such as quality shading, cream-skimming, or even the induced demand of services (moral risk)?

Some scholars and policy analysts argue that the market per se is not well suited to public services provision because in some areas, such as health and even education, many market failures can exist, namely:

1   Failure of competition,
2   Negative externalities,
3   Information asymmetry,
4   Insufficient provision of public services,
5   Service scarcity,
6   Market uncertainty, and
7   Monopoly or oligopoly formation.

Thus, the question becomes whether the traditional paradigm that the government acts in the public interest is true or if politicians or, to some extent, public officials pursue their own private interests (Mueller 2003; Hindriks and Myles 2006). Further, we should evaluate if it is possible to determine whether the government can guarantee its social functions in an entrepreneurial environment and how to avoid the distortion of the public service ethos. A creative solution must be proposed in sectors that require constant and persistent supervision and regulation. Further, a balance must also be reached between efficient public spending and safeguarding citizens' basic rights, namely regarding access to education and health.

The New Public Management in Healthcare

The increasing costs of healthcare delivery led to different political and administrative approaches aimed at preserving the core values of the welfare state. A recent report by the Organization for Economic Co-operation and Development (OECD) and the European Union (EU) (OECD/EU 2018) states clearly that health expenditure was growing at its fastest after the financial crisis. Moreover, the lack of responsiveness to public preferences and the under-provision of public goods (e.g., waiting lists for surgery) questioned the extent and capacity of public providers to deliver healthcare. Note that government failures in delivering important social goods are particularly difficult to accept in modern societies. Equity and fairness, that is, everyone should have access to healthcare according to clinical need, are important social goals. Therefore any healthcare reform should be evaluated insofar as these values are concerned (Daniels et al. 1996). Balancing efficiency (and the value-for-money) with equity (fair equality of opportunity) is a major political challenge in modern societies because citizens are more critical regarding the responsiveness of the healthcare system (Figure 9.1).

Healthcare has traditionally been delivered in many countries through public organizations that are expected to redress the imbalance that may otherwise occur in the distribution of health (Arrow 1963b). The search for equity in healthcare access and distribution was the main goal of public providers after World War II. The British National Health Service is a good example of such an organization. In recent decades, the costs of healthcare, including essential public health functions, have increased steadily due to biomedical research (e.g., genetics, assisted reproduction, oncology), emerging diseases (e.g., AIDS), medical malpractice, and increased life expectancy. Further, increasing efficiency has become another driver of most healthcare systems.

The successive reforms in the healthcare systems of developed countries have a common fact: maximizing efficiency is considered as important as guaranteeing adequate performance levels in the access to and quality of healthcare (OECD

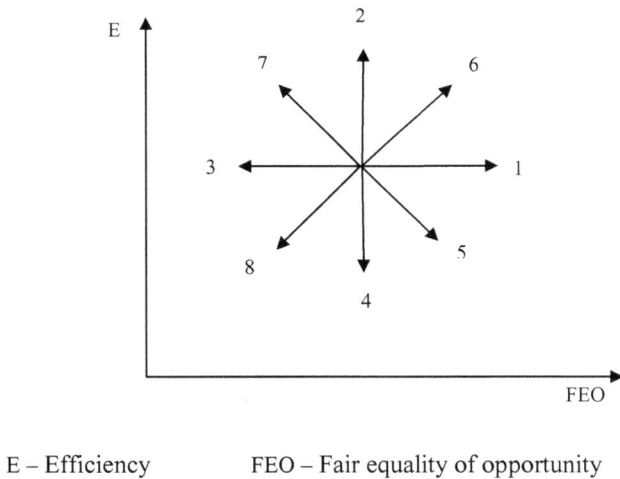

E – Efficiency   FEO – Fair equality of opportunity

    1.   ↑FEO ≈E (increase in FEO keeping E constant),
    2.   ↑E ≈FEO (increase in E keeping FEO constant),
    3.   ↓FEO ≈E (decrease in FEO keeping E constant),
    4.   ↓E ≈FEO (decrease in E keeping FEO constant),
    5.   ↑FEO↓E (increase in FEO and decrease in E),
    6.   ↑FEO↑E (increase in FEO and increase in E),
    7.   ↓FEO↑E (decrease in FEO and increase in E), and
    8.   ↓FEO↓E (decrease in FEO and decrease in E).

Figure 9.1 Strategic Clock in Healthcare Policy.

2018). Besides these important drivers of the reform of healthcare institutions, liberal democracies resort to other criteria, namely the fact that the healthcare system should consider citizens' perceived needs. Responsiveness is then a fundamental factor of any healthcare reform in an attempt to incorporate citizens' expectations into the main features of the reform. Nevertheless, responsiveness, or rather the capacity to meet citizens' wishes, is normally confronted with the problem of information asymmetry due to the specificity of the economic good at issue. It is especially important that a distinction is drawn between fundamental needs and mere preferences. An adequate regulatory framework can effectively draw these distinctions if the rationale for prioritizing is fair and publicly accountable (Nunes et al. 2017).

Although there are important cultural differences between countries and while most healthcare systems try to guarantee the tools for increasing health outcomes, financial sustainability is a major problem to be solved. The main strategies to control healthcare expenditure have been to maximize efficiency, establish comprehensive models of prioritizing services, or implement user fees. Increasing taxes is usually not an option because of the high opportunity cost involved and the sacrifices imposed on other social goods, namely environmental protection or research and development. To promote cost containment, many countries have applied the rules and principles of new public management (Griffith and Smith 2014).

Indeed, in most developed countries, the government intervenes directly in structures that provide healthcare services. Moreover, the government is instrumental in the planning, regulation, and evaluation of these systems. Most healthcare systems have different functions, including investment, financing of services, and delivery of healthcare. All of them try to guarantee the tools for increasing health outcomes. However, some countries are engaging in market approaches in healthcare based on the assumption that if competition is promoted, efficiency and resource allocation are maximized. A clear distinction between the financing and delivery of healthcare is the paradigm of this entrepreneurial culture because evidence shows that integrated models (financing and provision of healthcare) are usually more inefficient. As this argument goes, the government's role is to guarantee access to healthcare services and regulate this kind of activity. In this vein, competing models of hospital management have been proposed in the public sector through the introduction of private rules in its core administrative framework. The main goal is to obtain a flexible structure in accordance with demand, supply, and economic rationality and therefore, to improve health outcomes. According to Rego et al. (2010)

> The command-and-control system was an integrated, centralized, and vertical system – a military-style command-and-control model of authority related to the traditional administrative and management model of social protection systems. However, the incapacity of the state to respond to the expectations of the population, together with the lack of economic and financial sustainability of the system, promoted the introduction of a set of innovative policies.

Indeed, the introduction of new management modalities in the public system seems to promote competition; the best solution largely depends on social, economic, and political constraints (Nunes et al. 2009).

The distinctive feature of this reformist wave is the functional split between the financing and delivery of healthcare, which are being progressively delivered by different organizations with very different cultural backgrounds (public and private, profit, and not-for-profit). However, Laugesen (2005) claims that some market reforms are more legitimate than others. Namely, the purchaser–provider split and managerial reforms have been more successful than cost-sharing and competition-based reforms in financing and provision. Indeed, changes in the traditional structure of public administration have been consistently proposed, especially in the management of hospitals belonging to public services through new public governance. The introduction of the private finance initiative (PFI) perspective, in which a private group delivers health services (including sometimes clinical services) on a contractual basis (Sussex 2001), is sometimes thought to be another way to increase value for money (Appleby 2017). Although there are important cultural differences between the American, European, and Asian countries and while the national origins of different managerial and regulative techniques do influence the provision of care, most healthcare systems face the problem of financial sustainability.

New public management has been introduced to different degrees to guarantee the economic survival of the welfare state. This can be summarized as follows (Khaleghian and Gupta 2005):

1   Creating a split between purchasing and provision using output-based contracts for which private and public firms compete (rather than input-based financing of public agencies alone);
2   Giving managers' greater autonomy; and
3   Experimenting with incentive payments and other ways of improving worker productivity.

As stated by Preker and Harding (2003) "with increasing frequency, autonomization and corporatization are being considered and applied to improve performance of publicly run health services, similar to recent innovations in organizational reform elsewhere in the public sector." A shift from the government by control to the government by contract is the paradigm of this entrepreneurial culture. This typically involves the introduction of market processes, privatization, decentralization, and changes in organizational structure. Managerial autonomy and the corporatization of public entities (to different extents) have been typical in recent decades.

This entrepreneurial culture may be associated with important market failures that should be corrected by regulatory agencies. As an example of the importance of regulation, market uncertainty, which is an important market failure in healthcare, should be addressed by regulatory agencies (Stern 2012). In healthcare, uncertainty is associated with a different set of variables, such as fluctuating demand in accordance with clients' needs. Nevertheless, better decisions will be made if a particular market is evaluated, and better knowledge exists insofar as the agents are concerned. In addition, customer sovereignty, a well-known principle of competitive markets, is limited in healthcare due to information asymmetry, and is a psychological vulnerability that undermines the decision-making process.

In this context, while the US health system has obvious differences in relation to European and Oriental models, it is interesting to emphasize Michael Porter's view that competition in the health sector needs to be clearly reoriented since the free markets did not achieve the desired objectives. According to Porter and Teisberg (2004), since the US health system is strongly competitive, it must be asked why it has failed to perform well in terms of both cost and quality. According to economic theory, prices tend to decline in a competitive environment, quality is improved, and innovation leads to new applications that are rapidly diffused in a particular sector of activity. However, this is exactly the opposite of what is happening in the US health system (Porter and Teisberg 2004).

Indeed, in most liberal democracies, government intervention in economic activities aims, on the one hand, to define (and enforce) the rules of competitive markets and, on the other hand, to determine fiscal policy. In the case of strategic economic sectors for the development of a country, government's direct or indirect intervention is authorized to safeguard the essential goods in question. That is, even admitting some deregulation in strategic sectors (Whincop 2001), this should be accompanied by the implementation of mechanisms of self-regulation or external regulation (e.g., in utilities). Classically, market failures were met through direct intervention by the government as a producer. Health is a good example of this. The creation of public health systems and the inability of the market alone to provide this essential good meant that production was mostly from state services. Further, there was an important symbiosis between financing, production, and control of the system. That is, the state regulated itself. Telecommunications and the electricity sector are other paradigmatic examples. That is, self-regulated production paves the way for *distant regulation*, where competition becomes a decisive factor in ensuring market efficiency.

Thus, the search for efficiency creates the need for robust regulation. When public healthcare systems face the problem of cost containment, structural reforms are inevitable. Splitting in healthcare delivery does not mean that public providers (in the sense of ownership) will be completely replaced by private providers. If the government is directly involved in the provision of healthcare, while it may compete with private providers, there is an intrinsic conflict of interest between the government as both a direct provider and a regulator. A clear framework for independent healthcare regulation is needed (Walshe 2003).

If it is true that there is sometimes excessive political accountability because ministers are held accountable for what goes on in individual hospitals, the rise of independent regulators may increase public accountability. This will leave more room for good political governance (Nunes et al. 2007). It is assumed that equity is an important social value, and therefore, any reform should be evaluated insofar as this issue is concerned. To accomplish this societal goal, regulatory agencies must progressively monitor the impact of an entrepreneurial culture with respect to the balance between efficiency and equity in healthcare. As stated by Richard Saltman and Reinhard Busse (2002), "regulation, as a central instrument of stewardship, must from this perspective similarly satisfy these two basic requirements calling for ethical and efficient state behaviour."

The objective of the economic regulation of a particular sector of activity is to correct the failures of this market, considering the specificity of the good in question. Economic intervention through the competitive market is legitimate to the extent that it seeks to correct government failures, given the inefficiency of state management of public services. Through economic regulation, the intention is to control the free operation of the market and restrict the activities developed in it. In this context, the emergence of independent regulation is inevitable. The creation of independent regulatory agencies (IRAs) that are specific and dedicated to each sector of activity is a distinctive feature of the regulatory state (Gilardi 2004). Although it is well known that efficiency can be maximized with an entrepreneurial culture, important failures do exist in this setting. Then, stronger mechanisms of supervision and control are needed in healthcare. More importantly, there is a need to reframe the objectives of regulation in this changing environment (Baldwin et al. 2011).

Conclusion

Most healthcare systems are confronted with important challenges due to increasing healthcare costs and the subsequent lack of financial sustainability. The convergence of various factors, especially the demographic transition, will create the need for considerable creativity to overcome the inevitable economic pressures that social protection systems will encounter. The introduction of quasi-markets in healthcare is a reflection of this evolution. Importantly, this reformist course should be properly supervised to protect important social values. An example of this transformation is the creation of the United Kingdom Foundation Trusts (not-for-profit and public benefit corporations) that have closer community links and are therefore more distanced from the government than other National Health Service bodies. That is, management models must be found that will not only incorporate the market rules but also allow the implementation of principles and values protected in modern societies, such as accountability or responsiveness in accordance with communities' interests.

The configuration and interrelationships in the health market emphasize that this new wave of administrative transformations in the public sector should jeopardize neither the achievement that represents the right to healthcare nor the results obtained by many healthcare systems, which are in accordance with the global vision of the World Health Organization.

References

Appleby J. 2017. Making sense of PFI. Nuffield Trust – Evidence for better health care. www.nuffieldtrust.org.uk/resource/making-sense-of-pfi.

Arrow K. 1963a. *Social choice and individual values*. John Wiley & Sons, New York, 2nd edition.

Arrow K. 1963b. Uncertainty and welfare economics of medical care. *The American Economic Review* 53 (3): 941–973.

Baldwin R, Cave M and Lodge M. 2011. *Understanding regulation. Theory, strategy and practice*. Oxford University Press, Oxford.

Bossert W and Weymark J. 2004. Utility in social choice. *Handbook of utility theory*, S Barberà, PJ Hammond and C Seidl (Editors). Springer, Boston.

Buchanan JM and Tullock G. 1962. *The calculus of consent*. University of Michigan Press, Ann Arbor.

Congleton R. 2004. The political economy of Gordon Tullock. *Public Choice* 121 (1): 213–238.

Cullis JG and Jones PR. 2009. *Public finance and public choice: Analytical perspectives*. Oxford University Press, Oxford, 3rd edition.

Daniels N, Light D and Caplan R. 1996. *Benchmarks of fairness for health care reform*. Oxford University Press, New York.

Daniels N and Sabin J. 2002. Setting limits fairly. Oxford University Press, New York.

Davis E. 1998. *Public spending*. Penguin Books Ltd., London.

Gilardi F. 2004. *Institutional change in regulatory policies: Regulation through independent agencies and the three new institutionalisms". The politics of regulation. Institutions and regulatory reforms for the age of governance*, J. Jordana and D. Levi-Faur (Editors), The CRC Series on Competition, Regulation and Development. Edward Elgar Publishing Limited, Cheltenham.

Griffith A and Smith D. 2014. *Under new public management: Institutional ethnographies of changing front-line work*. University of Toronto Press, Toronto.

Hill PJ. 1999. Public choice: A review. *Faith & Economics* 34: 1–10.

Hindriks J and Myles G. 2006. *Intermediate public economics*. Massachusetts Institute of Technology, Cambridge.

Hughes O. 1998. *Public management and administration*. Palgrave, Hampshire, 2nd edition.

Khaleghian P and Gupta M. 2005. Public management and the essential public health functions. *World Development* 33 (7): 1083–1099.

Laugesen M. 2005. Why some market reforms lack legitimacy in health care. *Journal of Health Politics, Policy & Law* 30 (6): 1065–1100.

Le Grand J. 2007. *The other invisible hand: Delivering public services through choice and competition*. Princeton University Press, Princeton.

Lipsey D. 2005. Too much choice. *Prospect* 117. www.prospectmagazine.co.uk/magazine/toomuchchoice.

Majone G. 1994. The rise of the regulatory state in Europe. *West European Politics* 17 (3): 77–101.

Majone G. 1997. From the positive to the regulatory state. *Journal of Public Policy* 17 (2): 139–167.

Mueller DC. 2003. *Public choice III*. Cambridge University Press, Cambridge.

Mueller DC. 2008. Public choice: An introduction. *Readings in public choice and constitutional political economy*, CK Rowley and FG Schneider (Editors). Springer, New York.

Mullen P and Spurgeon P. 2000. *Priority setting and the public*. Radcliffe Medical Press, Abingdon.

Niskanen W. 1994. *Bureaucracy and public economics*. Edward Elgar Publishing, Cheltenham.

Nunes R, Brandão C and Rego G. 2011. Public accountability and sunshine healthcare regulation. *Health Care Analysis* 19 (4): 352–364.

New Public Management in Healthcare 135

Nunes R, Nunes SB and Rego G. 2017. Healthcare as a universal right. *Journal of Public Health* 25: 1–9.
Nunes R, Rego G and Brandão C. 2007. The rise of independent regulation in health care. *Health Care Analysis* (15) 3: 169–177.
Nunes R, Rego G and Brandão C. 2009. Healthcare regulation as a tool for public accountability. *Medicine, Health Care and Philosophy* 12: 257–264.
OECD. 2018. *Spending on health*. Latest Trends. www.oecd.org/els/health-systems/Health-Spending-Latest-Trends-Brief.pdf.
OECD/EU. 2018. *Health at a glance: Europe 2018: State of health in the EU cycle*. OECD Publishing, Paris. https://doi.org/10.1787/health_glance_eur-2018-en.
O'Neill O. 2006. Spreading suspicion: The nature of trust and its role in society, and is there real evidence of a crisis of trust? A question of trust. *BBC*. www.immagic.com/eLibrary/ARCHIVES/GENERAL/BBC_UK/B020000O.pdf.
Porter M and Teisberg E. 2004. Redefining competition in health care. *Harvard Business Review* 82 (6): 64–76.
Preker A and Harding A. 2003. A conceptual framework for the organizational reforms of hospitals. Innovations in health service delivery. *The corporatization of public hospitals*, A Preker and A Harding (Editors). The World Bank, Washington.
Rego G, Nunes R and Costa J. 2010. The challenge of corporatisation: The experience of Portuguese public hospitals. *The European Journal of Health Economics* 1 (4): 367–381.
Saltman R and Busse R. 2002. Balancing regulation and entrepreneurialism in Europe's health sector: Theory and practice. *European observatory on health care systems, regulating entrepreneurial behaviour in European health care systems*, R Saltman, R Busse and E Mossialos (Editors). Open University Press, Buckingham.
Stern J. 2012. The evaluation of regulatory agencies. *The Oxford handbook of regulation*, R Baldwin, M Cave and M Lodge (Editors). Oxford University Press, Oxford.
Sussex J. 2001. *The economics of the private finance initiative in the NHS*. Office of Health Economics, London.
Tullock G. 2005. People are people: The elements of public choice. Part I – The theory of public choice. *Government failure. A primer in public choice*, G Tullock, A Seldon and G Brady (Editors). Cato Institute, Washington.
Walshe K. 2003. *Regulating healthcare. A prescription for improvement?* State of Health Series. Open University Press, Maidenhead.
Whincop M. 2001. *Bridging the entrepreneurial financial gap. Linking governance with regulatory policy*. Ashgate Publishing Limited, Burlington.

10 Regulation and Performance Improvement[1]

The healthcare systems of developed countries are currently confronted with important challenges due to the rise in healthcare costs and the subsequent lack of financial sustainability (OECD 2018). The convergence of various factors, especially the demographic transition, will require considerable creativity to overcome the inevitable economic pressures from the social protection systems. The introduction of quasi-markets and new public management in healthcare reflects this evolution. Further, this reformist course necessitates proper supervision to protect important social values (Griffith and Smith 2014).

Indeed, the lack of economic sustainability of healthcare systems in most countries and a higher demand for increased quality and safety of these systems have contributed to the development of regulation as a decisive factor for modernization, innovation, and competitiveness in the healthcare sector. The role of healthcare regulation has two essential aspects. First, it intends to guarantee appropriate competition, namely in the context of a quasi-market where different providers apply for public financing of their healthcare activities. The government by contract is the paradigm of this type of service, where the guarantee of the quality of the services offered is more important than the institutional nature of the providers. Second, economic regulation intends to correct the market failures in this sector which require constant and persistent supervision: information asymmetry, externalities, service scarcity, market uncertainty, and monopoly creation. Healthcare regulation also intends to safeguard the basic rights of the citizens, namely concerning the practice of cream-skimming or even the induced demand of healthcare that inevitably leads to overtreatment. As such, social regulation is an instrument that affirms the basic rights of the patients.

Rise of Independent Healthcare Regulation

In this changing environment, it is not surprising that healthcare regulations are increasing steadily in most countries (Rego et al. 2010). As suggested by Kieran Walshe (2003), it remains to be seen to what extent these regulations achieve their objectives, namely performance improvement and ensuring fair

DOI: 10.4324/9781003241065-11

competition. Moreover, there is some dispute regarding which conceptual framework for healthcare regulation is to be adopted because regulation is traditionally regarded as professional self-regulation in the healthcare sector. Self-regulation of physicians is important due to its impact on professional standards of care, from a social and economic perspective; however, self-regulation does not always achieve its goal of effectively supervising a professional practice. Although medicine has strict ethical and clinical standards, there are often crucial flaws in its internal mechanisms of control. Often, it is precisely the medical practice itself that should be externally regulated. Therefore, the need for regulating its social and economic dimensions extends well beyond professional self-regulation (Clarke 2016).

Regulatory capture (in the sense of the regulator being influenced in its decisions by a third party) is frequently at stake because the control of a professional practice by one's peers may lead to conflicts of interest. Further, the self-interest of the profession may preclude the effective judgment of deviant behavior. Healthcare organizations have weak internal structures of control. Further, professionals still have a great deal of influence in the promotion of a culture that resists managerialism. Nevertheless, self-regulation still plays a major role in enforcing the ethical and clinical standards of healthcare professionals and should be regarded as an integral part of the healthcare regulatory system.

In this book, Selznick's (1985) definition of regulation is followed: regulation of any social and/or economic sector is the "sustained and focused control exercised by a public agency over activities which are valued by a community" (Selznick 1985). This perspective clearly focuses regulation on the supervision and control of specific activities by a public authority even though action in the public interest is usually considered to be paramount. This conceptual perspective of regulation is in accordance with the changing role of the government in most modern societies. As Giandomenico Majone (1997) points out, this gradual change is a distinctive feature of the *regulatory state*.

This perspective of regulation should be distinguished from legislation *stricto sensu* because of its normative and prescriptive content (Vogenberg and Smart 2018). Although abiding by the law is an ethical and social imperative, regulatory legislation intends to oversee the relationships between different parties in a more general way. That is, the regulation is restricted to specific economic areas and, therefore, is different from a legislation in both theoretical and practical dimensions. Judicial decisions are important drivers in healthcare policy because there is always the possibility of legal recourse through an individual lawsuit. Still, there should be another set of tools to maximize the potential for fair decision-making processes in this setting.

These two perspectives are not mutually exclusive; some legal arrangements are always necessary to accomplish regulatory goals. For example, if responsive regulation is at stake, this is a global approach that considers both compliance (Kon 2003) and deterrence strategies. For example, assume that the best outcome is achieved by matching regulatory instruments to the specifics of the regulated organizations and the circumstances in which the regulation is carried out (Ayres and Braithwaite 1992), that is, both *command-and-control* and *steer-and-channel* modalities. Then, enforcement through the law is a necessary condition (although insufficient) for the regulation to succeed.

Nonetheless, healthcare regulations have some peculiar characteristics. The specificity of healthcare regulation comes from a set of drivers that are particularly stringent in modern societies. In most contemporary democracies, the equity of healthcare access is considered as a positive welfare right; any deviation on this principle is regarded as an unacceptable failure of the regulatory system. It is also necessary to abide by the accepted quality standards because the wide definition of health as a general condition of well-being makes excellence in healthcare an ethical imperative. Then, efficiency in resource allocation is essentially a viability factor that must be considered due to the high opportunity cost of any decision in this setting.

I suggest that in publicly financed healthcare systems, regulation can be defined as the *sustained and focused control exercised by a public agency over health activities with the goal of balancing equity and efficiency, thereby complying with specific quality standards* (Nunes et al. 2009).

Healthcare is valued not only by the community but also as a major social right. Then, perhaps a specific definition of healthcare regulation should include its major goals. This framework assumes that a specific set of values should also be considered while defining healthcare regulation, namely the foundational values of the healthcare system. Balancing equity and efficiency, which are the main dilemma of public healthcare systems, may be a specific goal of regulation. This conceptual perspective is also useful to determine whether the new regulatory models perform better with respect to the control of market and government failure, namely, in the establishment of priorities in healthcare (Stern 2012). Then, healthcare regulations can be reframed much more specifically than it has been in the past, when it was regarded as tantamount to legislation, to include both independent regulatory agencies (IRAs) and direct government regulators. In the past decades, a new perspective of regulation has been adopted by most modern societies. The core philosophical approach of this new perspective is the need to control different providers (public, private for-profit, and private not-for-profit) that compete for the same contract (Sussex 2001). This competition can lead to unacceptable consequences in terms of rationing healthcare like unjust discrimination of patients in need of access to healthcare services.

It is understandable why IRAs are increasingly important for effective healthcare regulation (Nunes et al. 2007). Gilardi (2004) defines non-majoritarian institutions' IRAs as "public organizations with regulatory powers that are neither directly elected by people nor directly managed by elected officials." Its independent nature (political, economic, and financial) gives IRAs considerable administrative capacity in the healthcare sector with legal powers of supervision and control (Box 10.1).

Box 10.1 Characteristics of Independent Healthcare Regulation

1 **Public Interest:** The main goal of healthcare regulation is performance improvement based on the public interest to protect a major social good (healthcare access is a social and political right in many countries). Promoting competition through market-like approaches is an important, though a secondary, objective.
2 **Authority:** The regulator is recognized as such by all the stakeholders, and there is a specific legal framework for its activity.
3 **Centralization:** Control, supervision, and monitoring of the healthcare system are centralized in one or more specific agencies to ensure the best regulatory outcome.
4 **Independence:** To produce the best regulatory outcome, the regulator is financially, organically, and functionally independent from the government and the regulated organizations. In this way regulatory capture is avoided and equal treatment is promoted.
5 **Regulatory Governance:** The regulator is an exterior entity with respect to market activities and should be accountable to society in a fair and transparent manner, specifically to the Parliament Select Committee on Health and other formal institutions.

Independent regulators are particularly welcomed in market-based approach to healthcare when public providers compete with private ones for public financing. The growing role of non-majoritarian institutions reflects the changing nature of policy-making in which the lack of credibility of democratic politicians undermines long-term strategies. The delegation of policy-making powers to IRAs is justifiable to enforce healthcare policies that would otherwise be difficult to implement. Following up on this argument, it is reasonable to assume that the government's role is to regulate the provision of goods that are socially relevant, such as healthcare. In other words, the *regulatory state* has the task of controlling what would otherwise only be market forces (Majone 1994). For example, an independent regulatory agency regulates both private and public hospitals, although it belongs to the public sphere.

Pluralistic competition among providers, often found in traditional purchaser–provider splits and free-market systems, is not intrinsically inconsistent with the principles of equity, efficiency, and responsiveness (Khaleghian and Gupta 2005). However, market failure can lead to unacceptable consequences in healthcare that require effective regulation. Managed competition is itself a function of regulation, both in principle and in the traditional healthcare policy sense of a purchasing strategy that balances the competing demands of payers and users.

However, independent agencies can go even further in the control of the system. Independent regulators can avoid potential negative consequences, such as unjust discrimination of patients who need access to medical services. For example, since the creation of the National Health Service (NHS) in Britain and elsewhere, unsurprisingly, direct government regulation through the direct intervention of public officials has played a major role in regulation. In vertical healthcare systems in which financing and provision are accomplished in a hierarchical manner, regulation is always integrated with the delivery of healthcare. Direct regulation is a fundamental component of integrated vertical systems (Baldwin et al. 2011).

If competition is accepted as necessary for the healthcare industry, independent regulation is potentially more effective than direct government regulation if the government itself is a player in healthcare delivery. It will be easier for direct regulators to be captured by the government through political influence and indirectly by financial constraints on regulatory activity. Financial autonomy, accrued primarily from fees raised by regulated organizations, is a distinctive feature of independent regulators; this is why direct regulators cannot truly behave like independent ones. In a traditional vertical system, the accountability of elected public officials can improve transparency and the social justice aspects of regulatory functions; however, when public hospitals compete with private ones for a government contract, independent regulation is the most effective way to guarantee that decisions are not politically undermined. When the regulator must make complex and difficult choices regarding prioritizing services to be delivered to the public, independent regulators are better suited to accomplish fair decision-making.

In summary, the institutional nature of the regulator is a determinant in the regulatory outcome. There are similarities between direct and independent regulation, namely the existence of a legal framework that guides regulatory activity, centralized activity over the healthcare system, and the pursuit of the public good, including ensuring equitable access to and quality of healthcare (Donabedian 2003). A comprehensive framework for good regulatory governance is instrumental and accountability arrangements are also fundamental (Nunes et al. 2009). In this way, IRAs in the healthcare sector can be regarded as the logical consequence of the assumption of a different approach to regulation where regulators must control both public and private providers (Box 9.2).

Box 10.2   Principles of IRAs' Regulatory Governance

1   **Goals of Regulatory Governance:** To increase the performance of the regulatory agency, assure its social responsibility concerning the search for the common good and ensure compliance with accountability arrangements in a fair and transparent way.

2   **External Controls:**

a)   Public Accountability: Explicit, public, and detailed procedures for evaluating the regulator with a full public report (use reports, performance reports, compliance reports, and consultants), global budgeting, fair grievance procedures (legal and non-legal), and adequate privacy protection (adapted from Daniels et al. (1996)).

b)   Democratic Accountability: Auditing by political representatives such as the Parliament Select Committee on Health or other political bodies.

c)   Other External Controls: External mechanisms of reporting, public disclosure of the processes and rationale adopted in regulation, external audits, financial accounting, and annual reports (published on the Internet) (Nunes et al. 2011).

3   **Internal Controls:**

a)   Self-regulation: Internal audits, ethical codes, and disclosure of directors' performance and remuneration.

b)   Board: Singular versus dual board, mechanisms of appointment to the board, mechanisms of salary control, and performance evaluation (adapted from Mallin (2018)).

4   **Strategy:**

a)   Responsive regulation presupposes that cultural diversity between regulated organizations justifies the use of discriminatory power. Because this model is based on contingency, hierarchical regulatory tools are fundamental.

b)   To effectively regulate organizations' practices, an evaluation of each situation is required, followed by an intervention with the appropriate regulatory instruments.

However, if it is true that in a regulatory state, healthcare is delivered by different organizations with diverse cultural backgrounds, it is also true that all of them should be accountable for their decisions. Control by regulatory agencies is instrumental in accomplishing this goal. In many countries, regulators are at arm's length from the government. The National Institute for Health and Care Excellence (NICE) and the Care Quality Commission (CQC) are good examples of this regulation modality in the United Kingdom (NICE 2002). The rationale behind direct and indirect government regulation, as well as independent regulation, is easily understandable. As stated by Richard Saltman and Reinhard Busse (2002),

the strength of entrepreneurial incentives makes it essential to have in place adequate regulation to "steer-and-channel" what would otherwise be only self-interested private decisions. . . . Regulation, as a central instrument of stewardship, must from this perspective, similarly satisfy these two basic requirements calling for ethical and efficient state behaviour.

Public Accountability and Sunshine Regulation

The complexity of the healthcare system necessitates that healthcare providers are held accountable. Doing so effectively ensures that the two essential objectives of the healthcare sector regulation are achieved, namely, to promote healthy competition among providers and to uphold important social values such as the right to information and the freedom of choice. Public accountability is essential to combat the threat posed by encrypted data and to publicize performance indicators for each healthcare organization. Evidence-based performance indicators (i.e., social, economic, and quality) are necessary to accomplish these objectives. For instance, a repercussion of a bad score may be growing waiting lists for surgery that can be more properly managed with accountability procedures. The term accountability within this context refers to the need to make the decision-making process in all stages of the healthcare system visible and transparent, as well as the method for achieving transparency. At all levels of the healthcare system, important decisions are made concerning the amount of and way that resources are used.

According to Norman Daniels, the way these decisions are made is informative for evaluating the fairness of a healthcare system (Daniels and Sabin 2002). Each citizen has the right to know the underlying drivers of the decision-making process and to be an active participant in this process. This partnership implies that information asymmetry is reduced through informed consent, although the patient–physician relationship will always be directed by professional values. Regulation can play a major role in this setting by guaranteeing that patients are informed of their clinical conditions and associated options. At a macro level, this relates to the concept of democratic and transparent processes and promotes the participation of the society who, in accordance with its unanimously shared values, has the wisdom required to decide on issues such as establishing priorities in healthcare and on other topics of social importance.

From a political philosophy perspective, the term *accountability* has two distinct, though related, aspects. Public accountability refers to the duty to involve both society in general and the citizen in decisions related to healthcare. Thus, healthcare organizations are obligated to provide data and indicators so that citizens can make informed choices (Daniels and Sabin 1997). Democratic accountability refers to the process by which healthcare institutions, whether government, hospital, or an individual provider, are accountable to society. This may involve submitting periodic reports, performing internal and external audits, or even justifying determined courses of action, for example, when the adoption of guidelines for clinical practice is at stake.

Accountability also refers to the principle of autonomy, not only at the individual level but also collectively; social autonomy refers to the institutions with (or without) democratic legitimacy and the promotion of the right to information of each and every citizen. There does not seem to be an alternative since in a pluralistic and democratic society, no manager can meet the expectations of every cultural group; this is an indispensable factor in promoting social cohesion. Thus, for example, when allocating resources for a clinical intervention that benefits a

balance between compliance and deterrence. This combined model is called *responsive regulation* (Ayres and Braithwaite 1992). Thus, a graded hierarchy of responses to noncompliance with the recommendations and instructions of the regulatory entity develops. This enforcement pyramid intends to develop regulators' capacity to adapt to the current circumstances (Figure 9.1). The adopted model is not static but rather dynamic, depending on various circumstantial factors. Responsive regulation presupposes that the cultural diversity between regulated organizations justifies the use of discriminatory power. That is, organizations are distinct and thus, should be dealt with in a differentiated fashion. Since contingency is the base of this model, a hierarchy in the use of regulatory tools is fundamental. It is not possible to consider standardized use.

To effectively regulate organizations' practices, an evaluation of each situation is required, followed by an appropriate intervention with the relevant regulatory instruments. It is possible then to grade regulation-measuring instruments as these tools should have more significant weight in financial, technical, and material resources when the organization's performance is weak. This notion is partly related to the concept of empowerment associated with regulation. An effective regulatory system should be developed with the purpose of improving the performance of organizations, with characteristics such as contingency and hierarchy contributing decisively.

Regulatory agencies resort to distinct mechanisms depending on the organization's performance and cooperation with regulatory authorities (Baldwin and Cave 1999). When there are signs of bad behavior that put compliance at

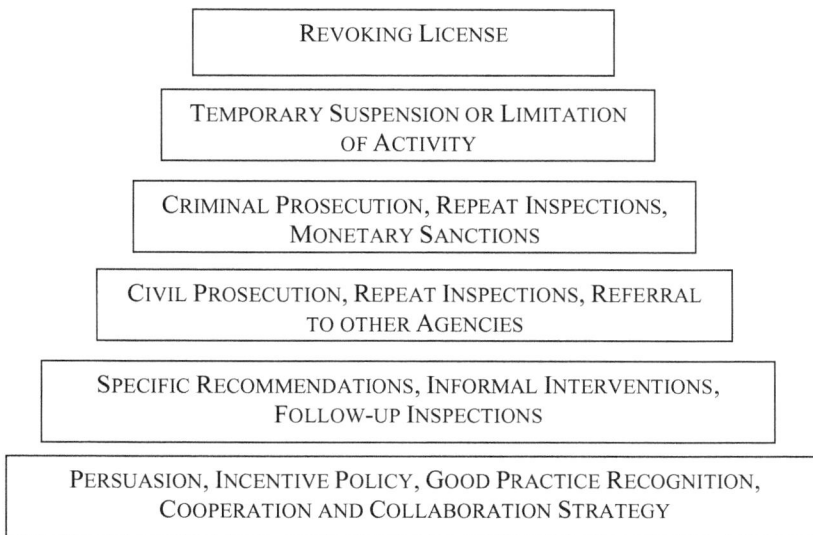

REVOKING LICENSE

TEMPORARY SUSPENSION OR LIMITATION OF ACTIVITY

CRIMINAL PROSECUTION, REPEAT INSPECTIONS, MONETARY SANCTIONS

CIVIL PROSECUTION, REPEAT INSPECTIONS, REFERRAL TO OTHER AGENCIES

SPECIFIC RECOMMENDATIONS, INFORMAL INTERVENTIONS, FOLLOW-UP INSPECTIONS

PERSUASION, INCENTIVE POLICY, GOOD PRACTICE RECOGNITION, COOPERATION AND COLLABORATION STRATEGY

Figure 10.1 Responsive Regulation – Enforcement Pyramid (Adapted from Ayres and Braithwaite (1992)).

risk, corrective measures should be introduced. Further, these measures should increase whenever milder measures seemingly lack efficacy. A lack of accountability necessarily leads to the reinforcement of regulatory instruments and therefore, of deterrence as a regulatory strategy. At the base of the pyramid, there are recommendations and guidelines indicating the standards to be followed by regulated entities. These will be for more frequent and general use in the regulatory process. It is fundamental that all regulatory instruments and the regulators' discretionary power are subject to some moderation by criteria such as prudence, transparency, and accountability (Whincop 2001). Further, the adopted procedures should be standardized and grounded for coherence and consistency so that the innovative nature of the regulator is not confused with a lack of determination. An integrated vision of the objectives of healthcare regulation and the means to achieve it is an important stimulus of regulatory activity. Responsive regulation depends on the systematic application of accountability arrangements so that it is possible to achieve effective sunshine regulation and allow the introduction of new governance models that prioritize citizens' interests.

An example of this evolution was the creation of the British CQC in April 2009. The purpose of this independent agency is "to make sure health and social care services provide people with safe, effective, compassionate, high-quality care and encourage care services to improve" (Care Quality Commission 2019). Most importantly, its values are the fundamental driver of its activity and the source of respect for society. This commission intends to achieve *excellence* being a high-performing organization, to be *caring* treating everyone with dignity and respect, to promote *integrity* doing the right thing, and to promote *teamwork* and an interdisciplinary culture. Again, note that the strength of any regulator is the prestige of its members and the excellence of its activity.

In both healthcare systems based mainly on the competitive market (such as the American system) and in public systems (such as the British NHS), the regulatory framework has developed considerably in the last few years, at least in part because competition exists almost everywhere. Indeed, the search for efficiency may easily cause healthcare services to malfunction so that regulation and supervision are even more needed. Different legal formats are acceptable with different degrees of independence from the government (Nunes et al. 2007).

Without regulation, the risk of providers' abuse is higher as they take advantage of their dominant position or market power, thereby providing lower quality services at higher prices. Therefore, what is really at issue is a paradigm change in which the concept of the state itself is questioned so that it is possible to implement statutory regulation in different sectors of the economy. Namely, in utilities that have significant social value. This evolution took place in the majority of Organization for Economic Cooperation and Development (OECD) countries in the past decades and is a central element in the development of a *regulatory state* (Majone 1994, 1997), that is, a regulatory state in which the central function of the government is to ensure that all citizens have access to needed services (e.g., healthcare, education, energy) and not necessarily a state that directly delivers these services.

However, the main issue is to determine whether regulation really works and how its main objectives may be achieved. According to Kieran Walshe (2003), four key characteristics are central to the nature and purpose of regulation:

1   Formal remit or acknowledge authority. In any system of regulation, the regulator has to have some kind of formal remit to regulate that is acknowledged by other stakeholders, most obviously the organizations being regulated. . . .
2   Centralization of oversight. Regulation represents a centralization of responsibility, power, and oversight in the regulator. . . . The regulator is regulating on behalf of others such as corporate purchasers, funders, consumer groups, individual consumers, and wider society, who cede some powers to the regulator in exchange for an undertaking, implicit or explicit, that the regulator will act in their interests . . .
3   Third-party accountability. As a result of the centralization referred to above, the regulator is always a third party to market transactions or inter-organizational relationships. In a market setting, the regulator is a third party to market transactions, providing a framework within which they take place and acting to constrain the actions of buyers and sellers. In non-market settings, the regulator is still a third party to the inter-organizational relationships and accountability arrangements. There will always be some kind of reporting, performance management or accountability chain through which an organization is overseen, but the regulator sits outside that chain of command or bureaucratic hierarchy.
4   Action in the public interest. . . . the process of regulation is intended to serve some wider societal goals, often established or expressed by the government.

Accountability (public display) and benchmarking (regular comparison) performance indicators provide a yardstick for competition between providers and lead to performance improvement. In general, there are two essential aspects of transparent and accountable regulation:

1   Public discussion of performance: The application of the principle of public accountability implies that the results of the benchmarking analysis are made public and scrutinized by society. In this manner, freedom of choice and competition in the healthcare system are ensured, as is citizens' empowerment.
2   Application of benchmarking: By comparing a set of performance indicators, it is possible to compare the economic, financial, and quality results of healthcare providers. The star-based rating of hospitals implemented by regulatory agencies is an example of this benchmark.

More than a performance principle, public accountability is the main driver of a new culture in the healthcare sector (Laugesen 2005). Independent of the degree of the state's intervention and the introduction of market rules, it needs to be applied effectively if the objectives of the healthcare system are to be fully achieved. Sunshine regulation depends largely on the implementation of this principle as it is not possible, without accurate data, to scrutinize the activity of healthcare providers. Thus, the existence of an appropriate and contemporary regulatory system is an instrumental factor in the global improvement of the healthcare system and consequently, of the population's health outcomes. A crucial aspect of sunshine regulation is the comparative benchmark analysis of healthcare providers, for example, the star-based rating system promoted by the British CQC and by the Portuguese Regulatory Authority of Health. This system exemplifies the hierarchization of relative quality that, according to the principle of public accountability, provides simple and objective information to the public (generally using four levels) on the global performance of the organization. In England, the CQC enacted the rating system. It was based on performance indicators reflected in the star ratings of NHS hospital trusts (Harris 2001).

Conclusion

Healthcare regulation has grown worldwide as an instrument of performance improvement (Crew 1999). Different regulatory approaches aim to overcome the diversity of government and market failures (Walshe 2016). The main goal of the regulation of public healthcare systems should be maintaining equilibrium between equity, effectiveness, and efficiency. Regulatory agencies should enact and enforce social as well as economic regulation.

Another driver of most healthcare systems is the prioritization of services. As suggested by Kieran Walshe (2003), it is reasonable to assume that many providers are "amoral calculators out to get what all they can." In complex healthcare systems that deal with many small organizations that are heterogeneous in nature and operate within a strong business culture, the struggle for economic survival can lead to unacceptable restrictions on patient access. In this setting, decisions regarding both direct and indirect limits of care will probably be left to market forces. Further, unjust disparities may arise in healthcare access. Although implicit choices were traditionally made by physicians and other healthcare professionals (e.g., selecting pharmaceuticals without any transparent procedure), modern societies welcome an explicit framework that is both fair and accountable.

The empowerment of a society can be only accomplished if citizens are actively involved in these choices. Accountability in the decision-making process can optimize equity and quality in healthcare. This is because easier access to performance indicators by a well-informed public reduces information asymmetry and empowers citizens to make accurate choices. Equity in access and quality in deliverance can be maximized in this way when resources are scarce. Equity (fair equality of opportunity) means that no one is unjustly discriminated against by the system, although a specific array of services can be withdrawn if there are relevant motives for such a choice.

In public systems within an entrepreneurial culture, supervision of the system is paramount to preserve the values embraced by modern societies. Then, a different conceptual framework is needed to address the flaws of running complex healthcare systems in a managerial sense. Distributive justice requires that in public systems, regardless of financing mechanisms and even under considerable resource constraints, priorities be established in accordance with the principle of public accountability; therefore, regulators have the social task of assuring that the rationales for limit-setting decisions are clearly accessible to the public. Sunshine regulation takes on relevance as by promoting publicly available performance indicators and open decision-making processes, it contributes directly and indirectly to the overall improvement of the healthcare system. Indeed, sunshine regulation facilitates the achievement of high levels of transparency in a decentralized network where entrepreneurialism appears to predominate. This transparency is necessary to overcome some of the market failures that are inevitable in the transformation of a vertical and integrated public system, in contrast to a regulatory state where systemic functions are disaggregated.

In conclusion, policy-makers must consider that the healthcare system involves different providers and that competition between different healthcare agents delivers the highest quality healthcare at the lowest possible cost. Adhering to the principles described here will uphold the core values of the welfare state, namely equity, solidarity, efficiency, and responsiveness. In this way, the fundamental human right to quality healthcare is honored at both the national and global levels.

Note

1 This chapter has contributions of previous published papers in the journals *Health Care Analysis* and *Medicine, Health Care and Philosophy* in coauthorship with Guilhermina Rego and Cristina Brandão.

References

Ayres I and Braithwaite J. 1992. *Responsive regulation. Transcending the deregulation debate.* Oxford University Press, Oxford.

Baldwin R and Cave M. 1999. *Understanding regulation. Theory, strategy and practice.* Oxford University Press, Oxford.

Baldwin R, Cave M and Lodge M. 2011. *Understanding regulation. Theory, strategy and practice.* Oxford University Press, Oxford.

Boyer R and Saillard Y. 2002. *Regulation theory. The state of the art.* Routledge, London.

Boyne G, Farrell C, Law J et al. 2003. *Evaluating public management reforms.* Open University Press, Buckingham.

Care Quality Commission. 2019. We're the independent regulator of health and social care in England. www.cqc.org.uk/about-us/our-purpose-role/who-we-are [Accessed 10 August 2019].

Clarke D. 2016. *Law, regulation and strategizing for health*. World Health Organization, Genève.

Crew M. 1999. *Regulation under increasing competition*. Kluwer Academic Publishers, Boston.

Daniels N, Light D and Caplan R. 1996. *Benchmarks of fairness for healthcare reform*. Oxford University Press, New York.

Daniels N and Sabin J. 1997. Limits to healthcare: Fair procedures, democratic deliberation, and the legitimacy problem of insurers. *Philosophy & Public Affairs* 26 (4): 303–350.

Daniels N and Sabin J. 2002. *Setting limits fairly*. Oxford University Press, New York.

Donabedian A. 2003. *An introduction to quality assurance in healthcare*. Oxford University Press, Oxford.

Gilardi F. 2004. Institutional change in regulatory policies: Regulation through independent agencies and the three new institutionalisms. *The politics of regulation. Institutions and regulatory reforms for the age of governance*, J Jordana and D Levi-Faur (Editors), The CRC Series on Competition, Regulation and Development. Edward Elgar Publishing Limited, Cheltenham.

Griffith A and Smith D. 2014. *Under new public management: Institutional ethnographies of changing front-line work*. University of Toronto Press, Toronto.

Harris C. 2001. England introduces star rating system for hospital trusts. *British Medical Journal* 323 (7315): 709.

Khaleghian P and Gupta M. 2005. Public management and the essential public health functions. *World Development* 33 (7): 1083–1099.

Kon J. 2003. *Understanding regulation and compliance*. Securities Institute Services, London.

Laugesen M. 2005. Why some market reforms lack legitimacy in healthcare. *Journal of Health Politics, Policy & Law* 30 (6): 1065–1100.

Majone G. 1994. The rise of the regulatory state in Europe. *West European Politics* 17 (3): 77–101.

Majone G. 1997. From the positive to the regulatory state. *Journal of Public Policy* 17 (2): 139–167.

Mallin C. 2018. *Corporate governance*. Oxford University Press, Oxford, 6th edition.

NICE. 2002. *Principles for best practice in clinical audit*, National Institute for Health and Care Excellence. Radcliffe Medical Press, London.

Nunes R, Brandão C and Rego G. 2011. Public accountability and sunshine healthcare regulation. *Health Care Analysis* 19 (4): 352–364.

Nunes R, Rego G and Brandão C. 2007. The rise of independent regulation in healthcare. *Healthcare Analysis* 15 (3): 169–177.

Nunes R, Rego G and Brandão C. 2009. Healthcare regulation as a tool for public accountability. *Medicine, Health Care and Philosophy* 12: 257–264.

OECD. 2018. *Spending on health*. Latest Trends. www.oecd.org/els/health-systems/Health-Spending-Latest-Trends-Brief.pdf.

Rawls J. 1971. *A theory of justice*. Harvard University Press, New York.

Rawls J. 2001. *Justice as fairness. A restatement*, E Kelly (Editor). Harvard University Press, Cambridge.

Rego G, Nunes R and Costa J. 2010. The challenge of corporatisation: The experience of Portuguese public hospitals. *The European Journal of Health Economics* 1 (4): 367–381.

Saltman R and Busse R. 2002. Balancing regulation and entrepreneurialism in Europe's health sector: Theory and practice. *European observatory on healthcare systems, regulating entrepreneurial behaviour in European healthcare systems*, R Saltman, R Busse and E Mossialos (Editors). Open University Press, Buckingham.

Selznick P 1985. Focusing organizational research on regulation. *Regulatory policy and the social sciences*, R Noll (Editor). University of California Press, Berkeley.

Stern J. 2012. The evaluation of regulatory agencies. *The Oxford handbook of regulation*, R Baldwin, M Cave and M Lodge (Editors). Oxford University Press, Oxford.

Sussex J. 2001. *The economics of the private finance initiative in the NHS*. Office of Health Economics, London.

Vogenberg FR and Smart M. 2018. Regulatory change versus legislation impacting healthcare decisions and delivery. *Pharmacy & Therapeutics* 43 (1): 34–38.

Walshe K. 2003. *Regulating healthcare. A prescription for improvement?* State of Health Series. Open University Press, Maidenhead.

Walshe K. 2016. Research, evaluation and evidence-based management. *Healthcare management*, K Walshe and J Smith (Editors). Open University Press, Buckingham, 3rd edition.

Whincop M. 2001. *Bridging the entrepreneurial financial gap. Linking governance with regulatory policy*. Ashgate Publishing Limited, Burlington.

11 Universal Access to Palliative Care

In contemporary societies, palliative care represents a different perspective toward facing both death and life. A different perspective of facing death due to the excessive technological character of modern medicine has resulted in an increasing dehumanization of clinical practice and a progressive distancing of health professionals from patients and their families. Palliative care, as active and global care, requires a significant increase in the affective dimension of the patient–physician relationship to promote patient follow-up, rather than trying to overcome death.

Palliative care is also a different way of looking at life. The concept includes a life with quality, life that anticipates death, and life over the long period prior to death. Hence, it is important to consider both the multi- and transdisciplinary nature of palliative care and the consequent implications for professional training. Great attention is already being given to this area of training; its teaching in medicine, nursing, psychology, and other healthcare professions is fundamental.

However, palliative care also has an appreciable scientific dimension with incursions into pharmacology and therapeutics with the aim of pain and other symptom control, in dignity therapy, in spiritual support, or even with respect to the specificities of the child and other especially vulnerable populations (Twycross et al. 2009). Moreover, palliative care has expanded beyond oncology care, which defined this type of care in the strictest sense; it is now fundamental in the treatment of cardiac, neurological, renal, or other terminally ill patients.

Historically, palliative care was born with the Hospice Movement in the United Kingdom and the seminal role of Dame Cicely Saunders at the St. Christopher's Hospice. This was the world's first purpose-built hospice in 1967. It was founded on the principles of combining teaching and clinical research with expert pain and symptom relief with holistic care to meet the physical, social, psychological, and spiritual needs of its patients and those of their family and friends. Palliative care provides a new perspective on health and disease. The ethics of care was a fundamental tool for the translation from curative to palliative medicine. Indeed, it is a new ethic that underlies this type of care, thus enabling medicine and other healthcare professionals to reconnect with themselves and the values they have always embraced (Beauchamp and Childress 2012).

DOI: 10.4324/9781003241065-12

From Chronic to Palliative Care

The increase in the average life expectancy reflects the improvements in health-care in most modern societies. In association with declining birth rates, an increase in life expectancy has contributed to the progressive aging of the population. This has created new healthcare needs related to degenerative diseases, sequels after an acute outbreak of a disease, dependence, and a greater survival in those with severe diseases. These types of conditions are the needs for which the hospitals are not prepared and to which primary care professionals and society are not able to provide an appropriate and timely response (Faull and Blankley 2015). Thus, beyond the legal and logistic creation of a network of integrated continuous care, it is important that there are trained professionals (in human and scientific plans) to make this type of care operational (Organization for Economic Co-Operation and Development 2005). The main areas should be developed with an operational context in mind as follows:

1   A national network of integrated continuous care;
2   Multidisciplinary/interdisciplinary care and assistance in chronic diseases and at the end of life;
3   Patient-focused communication and relationships;
4   Health education and autonomy promotion;
5   Health literacy and the special role of the government, third sector economy, social entrepreneurs, and professional organizations;
6   Patients with special care needs;
7   Training and support of informal caregivers; and
8   Audit, regulation, and quality control of long-term care and assistance-related services.

Indeed, society has the duty to protect the health of its citizens. This implies that the public healthcare systems should be organized to provide effective healthcare of recognized quality, especially when it comes to the most disadvantaged in our society such as the elderly, disabled, chronically ill, or people with high dependency, and people in other particularly vulnerable situations, such as terminal illness. In fact, one of the great dilemmas of contemporary society is the need for healthcare for this type of patients (Breitbart and Alici 2014). The nuclear issue is the quality of care and the way it is distributed among citizens, particularly in the field of geriatrics and gerontology. However, as the need for genuine intergenerational solidarity between the members of the community is emphasized, this solidarity must implicitly extend to the geriatric population. Thus, chronic care implies society's perception that this age group has its own characteristics with needs that differ from the younger population. In this context, the role of the family is essential. Further, the necessary infrastructure must be created so that elderly patients can be accommodated at home. Often, it is the elderly who have much to offer the family by participating in the education of young people and adolescents.

For implementation of community care, it is important that health authorities determine the individual needs of each patient and promote the necessary home care. Therefore, it is essential to periodically publish community health plans so that the population is an active agent in the decision-making process. Community care has two other particularly important dimensions in a modern society: a) the emerging concern with the creation of a network of nursing and care homes according to criteria of quality and humanization and b) the problem of promoting a true mental health policy through specific care for this specific population group (Kuebler and Heidrich 2007).

However, community and palliative care is not only dedicated to the elderly; in the broadest sense, it is dedicated to all chronic patients with irreversible diseases without any prospect of complete recovery and with substantial duration. Patients who need chronic care fall into one of the four major categories:

1   Autonomous,
2   Partially dependent,
3   Dependent, and
4   Highly dependent.

This typology refers to the spectrum of patient capabilities and the possibility of performing certain tasks alone or with third-party support. The goal of this type of care is the comfort and well-being of the chronic patient (and for the most part, of the terminally ill patient) using a multidisciplinary healthcare team especially sensitized for this purpose. Social solidarity institutions will certainly play an important role as an appropriate vehicle for welcoming the most vulnerable populations.

Invariably, the issue is dependence on others and serious limitations in everyday life (especially in the development of social relationships) because of the necessary provision of continuous and formal care, besides informal care by friends and family. More than treating and curing, the intention is to take care of the patient and integrate them into their family and society (Organization for Economic Co-Operation and Development 2013). Thus, a multifaceted and multidisciplinary approach is essential. As far as possible, the chronic patient's independence should be promoted in consultation with the family and with appropriate domiciliary or institutional support. In turn, professional support should include physicians, nurses, psychologists, healthcare and social service technicians, and other specialized professionals (Ferrell et al. 2015). That is, what is at stake is the adoption of macro, meso, or micro policies that can help these patients live with their illness or incapacity. Remember that the way in which each person views the disease is deeply related to the subjective interpretation of the phenomenon of becoming ill and its impact on personal biography (Bramadat et al. 2013). Thus, society should use the healthcare system to help chronic patients lead a high-quality and self-fulfilling life, surpassing, whenever possible, the existing physical, psychological, and social limitations (Figure 11.1).

Community-based chronic and palliative care is now considered as an integral component of the right to access healthcare of appropriate quality (Nunes

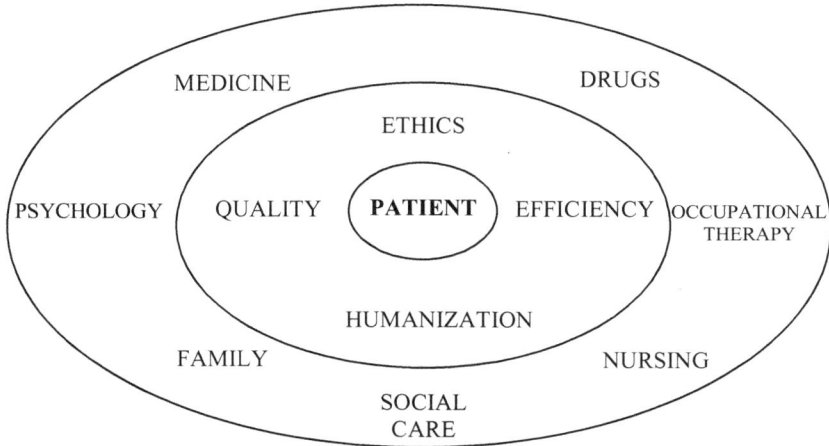

Figure 11.1 Chronic Patient: Expansion of the Quality of Life.

et al. 2017). Besides preventive health strategies, there is also a question of promoting home-based care so that people can stay in their homes whenever possible. Note that the concept of primary healthcare underlying the Alma Ata Declaration covers both community care and the curative intervention of the general practitioner. To truly facilitate community intervention, it is essential to both prioritize healthcare workers who provide home support and determine the real needs of the dependent populations. Competition between the public system, private initiatives, and the third sector can provide users with greater flexibility of choices and increase their satisfaction and well-being. The benefits to the community can be enhanced by more efficient management of human and material resources.

From a social perspective, chronic care must be prioritized for several reasons. On the one hand, the patients requiring this type of care (elderly person, chronic patient, mentally ill, and others) do not have the same claim capacity of young people or adults (Burlá et al. 2014). On the other hand, it was traditionally the family (especially women) who provided this care to their relatives (informal care sector). However, with the current social mobility coupled with an increasing role of women at professional levels, the number of chronically ill and elderly people living in isolation has become progressively higher. Moreover, there is a progressive disintegration of the traditional nuclear family. In this field, the existence of some gender inequality should be noted. Women, on average, have a longer life expectancy than men; the former relatively benefit from less informal care since they are precisely the individual who provides this care to their husband or partner. This fact refers to the importance of chronic care, either institutional or home support, when the chronic patient is alone. This isolation is aggravated by the fact that there is a decrease in the birth rate with a consequent decrease in the supply of informal care (at home and in health institutions).

However, the reversal of the demographic pyramid in many countries implies that different societies are now more aware of the need for chronic care, especially the crucial role of the family. A priori, it is up to the government to provide conditions for families so that they can adequately accommodate the elderly; direct support should not be excluded from households that do not have the resources to do so (cash for care). Nonetheless, the need to create a network of infrastructures and qualified professionals to treat and care for this type of patient is being progressively assumed by different healthcare systems. The proposal to create a national network of chronic healthcare in each country, and sometimes at the supranational level, aims to reverse this situation and articulate the provision of this care within the hospital and primary care networks, thus integrating it de jure into the healthcare system. A distinctive feature of this type of service is the need for effective coordination between different government departments, including the ministries of health and labor, and the social security system. On the one hand, this palliative care system is intended to promote social rehabilitation and reintegration; on the other hand, it promotes and maintains the quality of life for patients even in irreversible and terminal situations.

Thus, it is important to promote and regulate community centers, day care centers, and nursing homes, despite the home support required in particular circumstances. For example, in the United Kingdom, strict control is exercised by regulatory authorities over nursing and long-term care homes. There is even a specific agency, the Care Quality Commission, to regulate the provision of care at this level; that is, the different types and institutions of continuous care, namely nursing and long-term care homes, and residential family centers. This commission controls activities as distinct as medical care, the privacy conditions of the elderly, existing hotel conditions, or even the humanization of auxiliary staff, with sufficiently strong sanctioning powers to withdraw or suspend the operator's license (Care Quality Commission 2019). Issues such as the quality of care or humanization in patient–physician relations are considered of utmost importance, given the nature of chronic care.

Through the creation of a range of chronic and palliative care services, the intention is to provide the best care possible to people with loss of functionality or in a situation of dependency at any age and regardless of the cause of disability, including terminally ill patients. Patients and families have different needs; there are, for example, patients with low to intermediate complexity, intermittent complexity, and high complexity needs who tend to have persistent needs. For this purpose, different typologies of basic chronic care units should be created according to each type of specific situation:

1   In-patient units: convalescence units, medium-duration and rehabilitation units, long-term care units, and maintenance, palliative care units;
2   Hospital teams: discharge management teams, in-patient support teams in palliative care;

3   Outpatient units: day unit and promotion of autonomy; and
4   Domiciliary teams: integrated continued care and community support teams
     in palliative care.

In this integrated context, palliative care must be implemented effectively. According to the World Health Organization (WHO) (2013),

> Palliative care is an approach that improves the quality of life of patients and their families facing the problem associated with life-threatening illness, through the prevention and relief of suffering by means of early identification and impeccable assessment and treatment of pain and other problems, physical, psychosocial and spiritual. Palliative care:
>
>   1 Provides relief from pain and other distressing symptoms,
>   2 Affirms life and regards dying as a normal process,
>   3 Intends to neither hasten nor postpone death,
>   4 Integrates the psychological and spiritual aspects of patient care,
>   5 Offers a support system to help patients live as actively as possible until death,
>   6 Offers a support system to help the family cope during the patient's illness and in their own bereavement,
>   7 Uses a team approach to address the needs of patients and their families, including bereavement counselling if indicated,
>   8 Will enhance quality of life, and may positively influence the course of illness,
>   9 Is applicable early in the course of illness, in conjunction with other therapies that are intended to prolong life, such as chemotherapy or radiation therapy, and includes those investigations needed to better understand and manage distressing clinical complications.

Palliative care is active and global care that is provided to patients whose affliction does not respond to curative treatment with the aim that the patient and their family obtain the best possible quality of life (Twycross and Wilcock 2007). Professional support is crucial and should include physicians, nurses, psychologists, and healthcare and social service technicians specifically qualified for this duty. These concerns have facilitated the creation of a national palliative care network within the framework of a chronic care network. In the case of large countries such as the United States of America, India, and Brazil, networks at each state level are suggested, although interconnected with the networks of the other states. Within the framework of a national palliative care program, care may be provided within the hospital, health centers, or chronic care networks. However, there may be an advantage to the creation of a specific network in full articulation with the aforementioned networks.

A major concern is the need for care for terminally ill patients (Gordon 2015). In addition, in these circumstances, quality, equity, and accessibility to this type of care require more reflection. In fact, since the 1990s, the WHO has recognized palliative care as an integral part of the fight against cancer. Today, it extends to the treatment of chronic respiratory diseases, cardiac diseases, human immunodeficiency virus/acquired immune deficiency syndrome (HIV/AIDS), chronic degenerative neurological diseases, chronic renal failure, and other long-term chronic illnesses (Addington-Hall and Higginson 2011).

A national program encompassing palliative care should be implemented by recognizing the importance of this type of care (Box 11.1). This involves the creation of not only hospital palliative care teams but also community-centered palliative care units with emphasis on the articulation between domiciliary teams and in-patient units.

Box 11.1   Principles for a National Program on Palliative Care

1   **Principles**: a) Defend the right of terminally ill patients to access the full range of palliative care and b) protect incurable patients' right to make their own choices in the final stages of life (Nunes and Rego 2016).
2   **Recipients**: Patients who cumulatively have no prospect of curative treatment, rapid disease progression and limited life expectancy, intense suffering, and problems and needs with difficult resolution that require specific, organized, and interdisciplinary support. It is estimated that every thousand patients per million inhabitants will need differentiated palliative care per year (Rego et al. 2018).
3   **Essential components**: relief of symptoms, psychological, spiritual, and emotional support, family support, support during mourning, and interdisciplinary care (Rego and Nunes 2016).

The government must then promote domiciliary palliative care within primary healthcare, besides cancer hospitals and other healthcare facilities. Thus, good-quality medicine, an essential component of chronic and palliative care, must be based on both social support networks (which potentiate the resources of the dependent patient) and the family, which is the core element of any society. That is, humanization of health is a task that concerns all sectors of society; healthcare professionals have the responsibility to exercise their profession with the conviction that they deal with particularly vulnerable human persons.

However, the existence of networks with these characteristics, namely a national network of integrated care, should not prevent effective integration and coordination between primary, secondary, and tertiary care services (vertical articulation). From the citizens' perspective, the existence of such a network should be seen as an agent that facilitates movement at a certain level (horizontal articulation) and never as a sealed zone of the system which is difficult to access or transition. From a functional perspective, the network organization allows better knowledge of both public financing and scheduling healthcare services for the citizens' care. Moreover, a national network of integrated care should predict the plausibility of a wide range of healthcare providers in this field, for example:

1   Public entities with administrative and financial autonomy;
2   Private sector, for profit;
3   Private sector, not for profit/third sector; and
4   Healthcare centers.

Thus, accessing the network of chronic care should be done through the guidance provided by the hospital in which the patient is hospitalized or the healthcare center in which they are registered (Buchbinder and Shanks 2007).

Education for Palliative Care

The essential objective of palliative care education and training is for the professional to acquire knowledge in this field and become endowed with the skills and abilities for a more dignified and competent exercise of the palliative care profession (Billings et al. 2001). Professionals should also be adequately informed about the basic precepts of palliative care so that its practice unfolds according to the principles that guide this professional area. Further, specific training is intended to contribute to a better overall provision of community services by encouraging universal access to quality palliative care for all patients who may benefit from this type of intervention. Faced with the evolution of contemporary societies, mainly the existence of different perceptions of the phenomenon of death and the recognition of the existence of limits to medical intervention, a new approach to terminal illness has emerged, that is, palliative care, as an imperative of any modern and inclusive society (Cheatham 2015). The nuclear issue is the quality of care and the way in which it is distributed among citizens. Palliative care entails the societal perception that terminally ill patients have their own characteristics and needs that differ from other types of patients (Cherny et al. 2015).

Palliative care is intended for all types of patients (even children) with chronic illnesses, including patients with irreversible afflictions without any prospect of complete recovery and of substantial duration. The objective of palliative care is to provide comfort and well-being to chronic patients (and a fortiori, to terminally ill patients) using a multidisciplinary health team (Gawande 2014). Education and training are crucial for achieving this goal. Invariably, what is at stake is dependence on third parties and serious limitations in daily life (especially regarding social relationships) regarding providing chronic and formal care, and informal care by friends and family as a necessary component of this type of care. More than treating and curing, the objective is to take care of the patient and integrate them into the family and society. Therefore, a multifaceted and multidisciplinary approach is required. By creating different modalities of palliative care, the intention is to provide the best care possible to people with loss of functionality or in a situation of dependency at any age, regardless of the cause or degree of disability.

For adequate implementation of palliative care, it is vital to have education (pre- and postgraduate) and professional training at a differentiated level and according to a curriculum that has received international consensus (Stanford University 2019). Specifying the objectives of palliative care teaching and learning is perhaps the most important task in the organization of teaching and learning. The program content, methods, and materials necessary to achieve these objectives will be developed from this organization. The goal is to help students learn to achieve these objectives. Thus, from a cognitive perspective, the pedagogical objectives should include an attempt to increase professional sensitivity to the importance of palliative care in the context of terminal illness, promote critical reflection on personal, professional, and societal values in general, promote patient and family autonomy, identify clinical principles underlying decision-making, and allow a critical and systematic approach to decision-making in the clinical setting. Another aim should be to help the student acquire the necessary knowledge in understanding the grief and dealing with anger regarding chronic and terminal patients, especially with the concerns about the psychological and emotional dimensions of a patient with a terminal disease. In the conceptual plan, the aims should be the acquisition and knowledge of the core concepts in these areas and in the different types of psychological interventions in palliative care (Kübler-Ross 2014).

However, besides cognitive goals, the acquisition of behavioral goals is also important, that is, those regarding a specific interaction in the context of care. For example, the professional should know how to overcome the gap between theory and practice or that they have sufficient flexibility to accept the human condition at the end of life. It may be a question of learning to listen carefully and promoting respect for the patient's autonomy. There are some barriers that must be overcome in the palliative care teaching and learning process, such as: a) justification for the adoption of one theory over another and b) the problem of the affective detachment that death and dying sometimes evokes. According to the European Association for Palliative Care (2019), certain basic skills must be acquired through palliative care education and training, as noted below:

1 Apply the core constituents of palliative care in the setting where patients and families are based,

2 Enhance physical comfort throughout patients' disease trajectories,

3 Meet patients' psychological needs,

4 Meet patients' social needs,

5 Meet patients' spiritual needs,

6 Respond to the needs of family carers in relation to short-, medium- and long-term patient care goals,

7 Respond to the challenges of clinical and ethical decision-making in palliative care,

8 Practice comprehensive care co-ordination and interdisciplinary teamwork across all settings where palliative care is offered,

9 Develop interpersonal and communication skills appropriate to palliative care, [and]

10 Practice self-awareness and undergo continuing professional development.

Another essential objective is to teach the professional to be an active partner in learning by using different models of logical reasoning that stimulate critical reflection on the fundamental questions (Knutzen et al. 2021). In addition, the affective/emotional dimension in the relationship with patients, colleagues, and other health professionals should not be overlooked, especially when communicating bad news (Hagerty et al. 2005). Expectedly, this dimension is the least examined part of palliative care teaching. Being subjective par excellence, it becomes difficult to measure; still, it is possible to evaluate the position that each student may take in certain circumstances through discussions of problem cases.

From another perspective, it is perhaps a question of stimulating certain virtues that traditionally belong to the sphere of healthcare professionals (Quill and Miller 2014), for example, compassion, patience, and/or availability. This approach presupposes that some essential values are shared by all students and that there is a consensual hierarchy of such values. However, there is no doubt today that the fight against dehumanization is to improve human relationships or at least to combat the constant erosion of the healthcare system over the student in their positive attitude in the face of human suffering (Freeman 2015).

The affective and behavioral dimensions of palliative care students can be explored, particularly at the level of attitudes, considering different archetypes of learning (Van Aalst-Cohen et al. 2008). These techniques allow teaching and learning to be self-motivated and directed at both solving concrete problems and acquiring skills. Further, interaction, responsibility, and collaboration with colleagues are encouraged. By forming teams, especially in a multi- and transdisciplinary context, one learns better because in the effort to teach a colleague, interdependence is developed. These groups are preferably heterogeneous and randomly constituted and can be maintained throughout the teaching period.

Regardless of the strategy followed, it should be considered that healthcare professionals have a particular social responsibility by the way in which their activity enriches the debate on social values and the choices of a society. There should be a clear distinction between palliative care teaching for pregraduate students and those who wish to acquire more solid knowledge in this field, possibly for the purpose of an academic or professional career (specialization). While the first type should be considered mandatory, the second type is optional according to the interest shown by each student. In any case, the teaching of palliative care should be organized in the following teaching formats: a) theoretical classes (lectures on defined subjects); b) seminars (prepared and oriented discussion of specific topics); and c) group work (analysis and problem solving with encouragement and coordination of teachers and with the active participation of students), presentation by students of problem cases, and in-service training in the context of care. Promoting soft skills is paramount in all formats.

Thus, there is a complementarity between these different varieties of teaching and learning. The teaching of theoretical themes seems to favor more complete acquisition of knowledge besides its consolidation. This allows its functional integration with the lived experiences of each student's professional life. Teaching through seminars and group work concretizes the reflection previously made, allowing for the appreciation and broad discussion of paradigmatic problem cases. Besides problem cases concerning exotic, rare, and highly controversial situations, cases are also presented concerning frequent situations of everyday life. Educational approaches centered on real problem cases have proven themselves as important learning tools for palliative care, especially when the target public is a group of professionals with some degree of differentiation. These different strategies prove that cognitive data can be taught and comprehended. In addition, the development of competence in behavior and its relational dimension can be perceived through the referred methods, although it is more difficult (Field et al. 2001).

On a global scale, teaching palliative care is in accordance with universal priorities in the education and health sciences. Indeed, palliative care has the potential to stimulate the education systems of most countries to foster high-quality and inclusive lifelong learning for all and to change the way people face death and dying from a human rights perspective. In addition, inter-sector cooperation between the education and health sectors can be promoted through:

1   Promotion of the development of advanced practice in palliative care service organization and delivery;
2   Creation of leaders in palliative care;
3   Enhancement of scholarship skills;
4   Fostering critical approaches to evidence review and knowledge management;
5   Development of advanced skills in research design, practice, and dissemination; and
6   Acquisition of a critical understanding of policy issues affecting service development in specific settings.

To accomplish these goals, it is fundamental to empower learners to be creative and responsible global citizens. This is because since palliative care is a responsible way to approach citizenship in a fair and universally accepted way, thus contributing decisively to a true capacity-building strategy. Palliative care may clearly support inclusive social development and foster intercultural dialogue. By advocating accepted and universal ethical principles, palliative care fuels the promotion of a compassionate human relationship, autonomous and responsible decision-making at the end of life, and a fair and equitable society in accordance with universal principles of justice.

The values inherent to palliative care promote freedom of expression and freedom of choice. International scientific cooperation, namely through global networks in this field, will contribute to more sustainable development. Only well-informed citizens who are perfectly aware of their rights and duties can promote the need to protect the commonwealth of life. In addition, with this approach, gender equality will be promoted because it is well known that women are frequently discriminated against in healthcare access (Nunes 2020).

Moreover, palliative care teaching and implementation is in agreement with the United Nations Sustainable Development Goals, as defined in "Transforming Our World – the 2030 Agenda for Sustainable Development." At least four of these goals are regarding palliative care: a) "Goal 3: Ensure healthy lives and promote well-being for all people at all ages"; b) "Goal 4: Ensure inclusive and equitable quality education and promote lifelong learning opportunities for all"; c) "Goal 5: Achieve gender equality and empower all women and girls"; and d) "Goal 16: Promote peaceful and inclusive societies for sustainable development, provide access to justice for all, and build effective, accountable and inclusive institutions at all levels" (United Nations 2019).

Indeed, issues such as extreme poverty, halting the spread of HIV/AIDS, combating the COVID-19 pandemic, or providing universal primary education must be included in palliative care education and implementation because its principles and methods have the same primary goal of the promotion of human rights of the most vulnerable people. Indeed, the promotion of human rights and human dignity has several dimensions, one of which is the promotion of death with dignity. Education for values, including human rights, gender discrimination, inclusion of the elderly, and autonomy of the person (i.e., through the living will) is a specific endeavor of palliative care education, especially in low- and middle-income countries (Nunes et al. 2015). International cooperation is an essential step in promoting universal human values, such as those present in the Universal Declaration of Bioethics and Human Rights (UNESCO 2005).

Palliative care education intends to promote human rights culture worldwide, assuming that healthcare is a universal right, that is, regardless of the level of development of a particular community, everyone should have access to an appropriate level of care. In addition, palliative care has the potential to contribute to the transfer of knowledge in this field because this type of care depends much more on a human and compassionate way of facing chronic and terminally ill patients than on sophisticated and expensive technology. Networks that can be created worldwide may strengthen the links between different higher education institutions and other partners that share the same humanitarian ideals, such as nongovernmental organizations. The main beneficiaries are students (bachelors, masters, and doctoral students); however, many other people may be enrolled, such as high-school students, teachers, and policymakers. The objectives of strengthening these links include the following three main parameters:

1   Promote human rights and human dignity at the end of life by promoting palliative care as a new conceptual approach for dealing with a dying person with full respect for their autonomy besides their family's values and beliefs.

2   Share worldwide palliative care education as a new and vibrant field that requires specialized interdisciplinary training, from both a professional and an academic perspective.

3   Promote high-quality research in palliative care with a special emphasis on its implementation in particular settings from a cultural, social, and economic perspective.

This trajectory should provide specific data on death and dying, namely for palliative care, with the potential to promote true changes in the cultural perception of death and in the organization and delivery of healthcare that promotes the creation of universal access to palliative care. Skills (including soft skills) are clearly and definitively enhanced in this area because students, academics, professionals, policy-makers, and citizens should be able to acquire the necessary knowledge in palliative care, especially in terms of the foundation of this practice and its relationship with healthcare professionals (Hockley et al. 2013). From a research perspective, students should acquire skills that enable them to perform high-level scientific research in palliative care (Addington-Hall et al. 2007).

Conclusion

In summary, the way people die is a thorough indicator of the level of implementation of human rights and equal opportunity policies in modern societies. This is the reason for an observable dual trend in most civilized countries. On the one hand, better healthcare systems have been developed and implemented with sophisticated technology and innovative pharmaceuticals. On the other hand, death and dying are also approached from a humanitarian perspective that has led to a worldwide palliative care movement (Okun and Nowinski 2012). In Europe, this movement began in the United Kingdom in the 1960s, but is now widespread in all member states of the European Union and in many other countries worldwide. Palliative care implies the assumption of core values, such as human dignity and human rights, as the main driver of any modern and civilized society. Therefore, society must promote the generalization of palliative care at home, in primary healthcare, cancer hospitals, and other health facilities.

Within this framework, there is now a consensus that palliative care should be taught, longitudinally, throughout in-service with ongoing and lifelong professional training in medicine and other health sciences. That is, there should be specific training in the pregraduation curricula of physicians, nurses, psychologists, and other healthcare professionals (Nicol and Nyatanga 2014). Further, there should be complementary teaching at the master's and doctoral levels for all of those who wish to deepen their training. However, academic education must be accompanied by appropriate professional training. Thus, professional associations should also recognize the importance of palliative care through the creation of professional specializations.

References

Addington-Hall J, Bruera E, Higginson I et al. 2007. *Research methods in palliative care.* Oxford University Press, New York.

Addington-Hall J and Higginson I. 2011. *Palliative care for non-cancer patients.* Oxford University Press, New York.

Beauchamp T and Childress J. 2012. *Principles of biomedical ethics.* Oxford University Press, New York, 7th edition.

Billings JA, Ferris FD, Macdonald N et al. 2001. Hospice home care working group. The role of palliative care in the home in medical education: Report from a national consensus conference. *Journal of Palliative Medicine* 4 (3): 361–371.

Bramadat P, Coward H and Stajduhar K. 2013. *Spirituality in hospice palliative care,* SUNY Series in Religious Studies. State University of New York Press, New York.

Breitbart W and Alici Y. 2014. *Psychosocial palliative care.* Oxford University Press, New York.

Buchbinder SB and Shanks NH. 2007. *Introduction to health care management.* Jones & Bartlett Learning, Burlington, MA.

Burlá C, Rego G and Nunes R. 2014. Alzheimer, dementia and the living will: A proposal. *Medicine, Health Care and Philosophy* 17 (3): 389–395.

Care Quality Commission. 2019. The independent regulator of health and social care in England www.cqc.org.uk/.

Cheatham C. 2015. *Hospice whispers: Stories of life.* SCIE Publishing, New York.

Cherny N, Fallon M, Kaasa S et al. 2015. *Oxford textbook of palliative medicine.* Oxford University Press, New York, 5th edition.

European Association for Palliative Care. 2019. Core competencies in palliative care: An EAPC White Paper on palliative care education. Prepared by Claudia Gamondi, Philip Larkin, and Sheila Payne. www.eapcnet.eu/Themes/Education.aspx.

Faull C and Blankley K. 2015. *Palliative care.* Oxford University Press, New York, 2nd edition.

Ferrell B, Coyle N and Paice J. 2015. *Oxford textbook of palliative nursing.* Oxford University Press, New York.

Field D, Clark D, Corner J et al. 2001. *Researching palliative care.* Open University Press, Maidenhead.

Freeman B. 2015. *Compassionate person-centered care for the dying: An evidence-based guide for palliative care nurses.* Springer Publishing Company Inc., New York.

Gawande A. 2014. *Being mortal: Medicine and what matters in the end.* Metropolitan Books, New York.

Gordon PS. 2015. *Psychosocial interventions in end-of-life care: The hope for a "good death", research in death studies.* Routledge, London.

Hagerty RG, Butow PN, Ellis PM et al. 2005. Communicating prognosis in cancer: A systematic review of the literature. *Annals of Oncology* 16 (7): 1005–1053.

Hockley J, Froggatt K and Heimerl K. 2013. *Participatory research in palliative care: Actions and reflections.* Oxford University Press, New York.

Knutzen K, Sacks O, Brody-Bizar O et al. 2021. Actual and missed opportunities for end-of-life care discussions with oncology patients. A qualitative study. *JAMA Network Open 2021* 4 (6): e2113193.

Kuebler KK and Heidrich DE. 2007. *Palliative & end-of-life care: Clinical practice guidelines.* Peg Espers Saunders Elsevier, Amsterdam, 2nd edition.

Kübler-Ross E. 2014. *On death and dying: What the dying have to teach doctors, nurses, clergy and their own families.* Scribner Publishing, New York.

Nicol J and Nyatanga B. 2014. *Palliative and end of life care in nursing.* Transforming Nursing Practice Series. Sage Publications Ltd, London.

Nunes R. 2020. Addressing gender inequality to promote basic human rights and development: A global perspective. *CEDIS Working Papers* 2020 (1). http://cedis.fd.unl.pt/blog/project/addressing-gender-inequality-to-promote-basic-human-rights-and-development-a-global-perspective/.

Nunes R, Duarte I, Santos C et al. 2015. *Education for values and bioethics.* SpringerPlus 2015. DOI: 10.1186/s40064-015-0815-z.

Nunes R, Nunes SB and Rego G. 2017. Healthcare as a universal right. *Journal of Public Health* 25: 1–9.

Nunes R and Rego G. 2016. Euthanasia: A challenge to medical ethics. *Journal of Clinical Research & Bioethics* 7: 4.

Okun B and Nowinski J. 2012. *Saying goodbye: A guide to coping with a loved one's terminal illness.* Berkley Books, New York.

Organization for Economic Co-Operation and Development. 2005. *The OECD health project – Long-term care for older people.* OECD Publishing, Paris.

Organization for Economic Co-Operation and Development/European Commission. 2013. *A good life in old age? Monitoring and improving quality in long-term care.* OECD Publishing, Paris.

Quill T and Miller F. 2014. *Palliative care and ethics.* Oxford University Press, New York.

Rego MF and Nunes R. 2016. The interface between psychology and spirituality in palliative care. *Journal of Health Psychology* 24 (3): 279–287.

Rego MF, Pereira C, Rego G and Nunes R. 2018. The psychological and spiritual dimensions in palliative care: A descriptive systematic review. *Neuropsychiatry* 8 (2): 484–494.

Stanford University. 2019. *End of life curriculum project. End of life online curriculum.* Stanford. http://endoflife.stanford.edu.

Twycross R and Wilcock A. 2007. *Palliative care formulary.* Pharmaceutical Press, Nottingham City, 3rd edition. www.palliativedrugs.com.

Twycross R, Wilcock A and Toller C. 2009. *Symptom management in advanced cancer.* Pharmaceutical Press, Nottingham City, 4th edition. www.palliativedrugs.com.

UNESCO. 2005. Universal declaration of bioethics and human rights. www.unesco.org/new/en/social-and-human-sciences/themes/bioethics/bioethics-and-human-rights/.

United Nations. 2019. United nations sustainable development goals. https://sustainabledevelopment.un.org/?menu=1300.

Van Aalst-Cohen E, Riggs R and Byock I. 2008. Palliative care in medical school curricula: A survey of United States medical schools. *Journal of Palliative Medicine* 11 (9): 1200–1202.

WHO. 2013. World Health Organization definition of palliative care. www.who.int/cancer/palliative/definition/en/.

12 Patients' Rights in Modern Societies

Over the past few years, health systems have undergone considerable progress, especially with respect to their management models. In fact, the resources that citizens provide for the health sector are already considerable in most countries. Therefore, the economic and financial sustainability of the system should be considered one of the top priorities of any society.

Nevertheless, generating efficiency in this sector to ensure its future viability cannot be an objective that is oblivious to the core values of pluralistic societies. Since healthcare access is considered a basic right, any structural reform of the health system must be based on the primacy of the human person along with fundamental rights (Nunes et al. 2017). Equity in access, nondiscrimination, and quality of care, among other factors, are the faces of a polyhedron that is undergoing constant evolution to adapt to the profound transformations in the health system (Buchanan 2000). Therefore, it is necessary to redefine the framework of patients' rights in healthcare services and to make this framework more robust in the face of resource scarcity demonstrated in all societies. In other words, it is important to ensure that every individual has the right of universal and equal access to the public healthcare system, to ensure adequate standards of quality, and to ensure the legitimate rights and interests of all users.

In contrast, the introduction of competitive market rules in the healthcare sector as a mechanism of efficiency implies that other realities, such as respect for freedom of choice in health facilities or guaranteeing the right of universal access to public services, should also be safeguarded. Thus, many countries have opted to create patient charters. In fact, patient charters should be considered the normative benchmark of the vast array of rights devoted to the patient and other users of the health system. These rights include rights both as a person and as a sick patient.

In other words, the principles, values, and rights enshrined in these charters should cover the generality of patients but also specific populations such as children, pregnant women, disabled individuals, and elderly people, who constitute populations that should be accorded special approaches so that their specific characteristics can be truly guarded. Moreover, promoting intense public debates on this theme contributes to a more just and equitable society (CIOMS 1997).

DOI: 10.4324/9781003241065-13

Democracy and Basic Rights

The enjoyment of basic rights by citizens is largely dependent on the evolution of many societies into liberal democracies, in which democracy and human rights have evolved concurrently. Therefore, democratic structure is a prerequisite for certain rights to be enjoyed by all citizens as a general principle of the rule of law, regarding individual self-determination, and the exercise of personal privacy and nondiscrimination.

In liberal democracies, credibility and legitimacy are necessary conditions for political actions to be ethically and socially justifiable. Therefore, adequate means must be found for political decisions to have the necessary substantive, and not merely formal, legitimacy. This legitimacy implies respect for the will of the people through adequate representation. In short, political action in (liberal) democracy must be guided by the concretization of different principles that are at the base of any modern and pluralistic society (Nunes and Rego 2014):

1   Responsiveness,
2   Empowerment, and
3   Accountability.

In democracy, the source of legitimacy that is substantive and not merely formal can come from two different sources. The primary source stems from the popular will expressed through the vote in the framework of clear and unambiguous proposals that are borne in specific electoral acts. This first source is the most widely used solution because it reflects the will of the majority. However, it has the disadvantage of relegating the opinions and perspectives of minorities to the background. Based on the rules of representative democracy, these minorities have more difficulty in making their voices heard. Representation has the enormous advantage of allowing adequate governability since elected officials are mandated to execute a program previously validated by voters. It is hoped that there is a huge congruence and even correspondence between the validated and the executed program (responsiveness), even though this is not always the case.

In this context, it has been suggested that as an alternative source of legitimacy, active and participative involvement of society and different social actors (empowerment) should occur. To be legitimate, the direct participation of society in collective purposes implies a broad base of support so that the absence of citizens' votes can be filled by an adequate, enlarged, and transparent representation (accountability). Greater participation in collective life is an expression of higher levels of citizenship and civic responsibility (Dworkin 2000). However, given the discreditation of the political system in many countries, it is not surprising that citizens distanced themselves from political life. Therefore, new forms of more direct democracy (e.g., rational democratic deliberation) are welcome, but should always be in balance with the representation through the activities of the represented parties to guarantee adequate governability.

Increasing participation through referendums is a prerogative of modern and civilized countries. These are legitimate methods that reveal the maturity of people (very common, e.g., in Switzerland). Rational democratic deliberation is an alternative to the decision-making process. Deliberative democracy was originally proposed by Joseph M. Bessette in 1980, who suggested that authentic deliberation (a mix of majority rule and decision by consensus) is a source of legitimacy when it comes from a direct process of decision-making by the citizens, which is a form of direct democracy (Bessette 1981). Another form is participatory democracy. In any case, this increased participation of citizens in collective endeavors is inevitable, especially in extreme situations in which elected political power not only is legitimized to make decisions but also seeks to avoid accountability for specific decisions (Arendt 1995; Habermas 1997). The transition from a traditional *bureaucratic state* to a *regulatory state* is partly because independent regulatory agencies (IRA) are used to implement unsympathetic measures to supplant politicians' inability to undertake such measures (Majone 1997). Indeed, it may seem a paradox that unelected agencies make hard social and economic choices. However, this paradox is only apparent because IRAs are directly accountable to the people through new modalities of accountability and responsiveness (Nunes et al. 2011).

However, the virtues of democracy are not confined to a single society and must be generalized at an international level. At the global level, there seems to be no better alternative to democracy for accomplishing peace, development, the rule of law, and human rights. Andrew Beddow, following Immanuel Kant's democratic peace theory, stated,

> Just as men must overcome this anarchic condition of injustice by establishing a civil state, states must institute an international legal order in the form of a federation of states submitting to a common adjudicative authority. Only then, can coercion become regulated in the international sphere and represent the omnilateral will of the human race, just as the state represents the will of its people. . . . Only a democratic world order, in which each state's population internalizes the costs of its own behaviour, can organize itself into a liberal world order in which states are regulated by law.
>
> (Beddow 2017)

Kantian perpetual peace rests on three main institutional evolutions (Caranti 2016): a) liberal democracies should evolve to full democracies with active citizenship and social participation; b) global governance arrangements should be promoted so that supranational institutions can be truly effective (the United Nations (UN) and the International Criminal Court are good examples); and c) freedom of circulation (or the right to visit) should exist to allow the mobility of citizens and their families (such as in the European Union (EU)).

The democratic regime is not only more ideologically virtuous in promoting the exercise of individual freedom, but it also increases civic participation of citizens with respect to collective goals, such as healthcare promotion. Indeed, several global studies have highlighted the role of democracy in improving health. Democracy, through popular representation and through the satisfaction of the basic needs of the populations, meets the desire of any human being to have an increasingly satisfactory quality of life in terms of access to health, education, and other essential goods, such as protection in old age or maternity (Nunes and Rego 2014). According to Bollyky et al. (2019), the

> Democratic rule, enforced by regular free and fair elections, appears to make an important contribution to adult health by increasing government spending on health and potentially reducing deaths from several non-communicable diseases (NCDs) and transport injuries. Conversely, autocracies that escape this general scrutiny, and do not have the same external pressures or support from global health donors to tackle NCDs and injuries, may have less incentive to finance their prevention and treatment, and seem to underperform as a result.

The Institute for Health Metrics and Evaluation (2019) also agrees

> that elections and the health of the people are increasingly inseparable. Democratic institutions and processes, and particularly free and fair elections, can be an important catalyst for improving population health, with the largest health gains possible for cardiovascular and other non-communicable diseases. Conversely, efforts to separate population health from elections and the other hallmarks of democracy might be less successful, especially as aid budgets are stagnant and countries' needs shift to non-communicable diseases, injuries, and adult health. This study suggests that democratic governance and its promotion, along with other government accountability measures, might further enhance efforts to improve population health.

There is a close link between democracy, global health, and human rights. Democracies clearly improve several aspects of peoples' lives, such as:

1   Life expectancy,
2   Health outcome,
3   Mortality rates (cardiovascular disease for instance),
4   Access to useful medicines (Simão et al. 2018),
5   Road deaths, and
6   Increases in government health spending.

Discussions about democracy today still incorporate the notion that we live in a global world (McLuhan and Powers 1989) which brings different people together through a liberal economic order that allows for free international trade. A global economic order that extends beyond borders implies cooperation between societies with different cultures, traditions, and religious or even political backgrounds. From a commercial perspective, the Belt and Road Initiative is an example of the way countries interact today (the starting point of the Silk Road Economic Belt is in Xi'an, China, and the endpoint is in Rotterdam, the Netherlands) (Jia and Wang 2019). In addition, with respect to healthcare access, this global geopolitical conjuncture should be considered, namely because it is well known that one of the great global challenges of the 21st century is climate change. Advanced democracies in this global economic order must realize that climate change is a central issue and that it will be vital to deliver an accelerated response to this dramatic evolution (Watts et al. 2018). Climate change is a challenge that involves all societies, democratic or otherwise. Its impacts on health and global health improvement should be carefully evaluated (Capon and Corvalana 2018). Therefore, there has been a global movement to decarbonize the economy, rebuild the environment, and substantially increase the marine protected areas to at least 30% of the ocean (combating heating, deoxygenation, and acidity of the oceans).

However, a priori, one may ask: what is the ethical basis of individual rights in a global society? (Sen 1999) In particular, the right to individual self-determination and the principle of respect for autonomy are framed in a context in which physicians and patients often have different visions of the individual and the common good. Typically, in pluralistic and democratic societies, citizens are more critical and demanding and do not accept the coercive imposition of any ideological orthodoxy. The very concepts of ethics and morals, besides their rationale, are not without controversy. Therefore, there is an urgent need to reach a consensus on the universal ethical principles. The Council of Europe's approval of the Convention for the Protection of Human Rights and Dignity of the Human Being, regarding the Application of Biology and Medicine (Council of Europe 1996) and by United Nations Economic, Social, and Cultural Organization (UNESCO) of the Universal Declaration of Bioethics and Human Rights (UNESCO 2005), aims to meet the perceived need to find an ethical minimum on a global scale and thus, offering better protection of patients' rights.

In addition, global ethical standards should consider the Universal Declaration of Human Rights as of December 10, 1948; the Universal Declaration on the Human Genome and Human Rights adopted by the General Conference of UNESCO on November 11, 1997; the UN Convention on the Elimination of All Forms of Discrimination against Women on December 18, 1979; and the Declaration on the Elimination of Violence Against Women adopted by the UN General Assembly on December 20, 1993. This list also includes the UN International Covenant on Economic, Social and Cultural Rights, and the International Covenant on Civil and Political Rights of December 16, 1966; the UN International Convention on the Elimination of All Forms of Racial Discrimination of December 21, 1965; the UN Convention on the Rights of the Child of November 20, 1989; the UN Convention on Biological Diversity of June 5, 1992; the Standard Rules on the Equalization of Opportunities for Persons with Disabilities adopted by the UN General Assembly in 1993; the UNESCO Declaration on Race and Racial Prejudice of November 27, 1978; the UNESCO Declaration on the Responsibilities of the Present Generations Towards Future Generations of November 12, 1997; the UNESCO Universal Declaration on Cultural Diversity of November 2, 2001;

and other relevant international instruments adopted by the UN, particularly the World Health Organization (WHO).

In summary, within this overall ethical and legal framework, the patient, as a person, enjoys the following fundamental rights:

1   Right to life,
2   Right to moral and physical integrity,
3   Right to freedom,
4   Right to freedom of thought, conscience, religion, opinion, and expression,
5   Right to personal identity,
6   Right to free development of personality,
7   Right to privacy,
8   Right to education,
9   Right to a standard of living that is adequate for the patient and the patient´s family,
10 Right to work,
11 Right to social security,
12 Right to health protection, and
13 Right to benefit from scientific progress and its applications.

These rights indicate that autonomy, information, previously expressed will, claims and complaints, access to health information, freedom of choice, individual privacy, nondiscrimination and non-stigmatization, spiritual support, primacy of the person over science and society, and equity in access and timely accessibility to healthcare are the pillars of a new health system. Patients' charters are useful tools for remembering these rights and should be implemented in every healthcare system according to the cultural specificities of a given society.

The Right to Self-Determination

The right to self-determination is closely linked to the principle of respect for persons (Beauchamp and Childress 2013). To be a full human person, anyone should have the opportunity to make choices regarding every aspect of their human life. Thus, the concept of autonomy refers to the perspective that every rational human being should be truly free and have the minimum conditions for self-realization. Free will is the natural condition of the human being due to its rationality and intentionality, which makes humans not only agents but also moral agents because they have the extraordinary capacity to decide in accordance with their ethical standards. Usually, although not always, the special vulnerability of the patient does not undermine this capacity. In addition, in a global culture, especially in the case of children, adolescents, or other persons with diminished mental capacities, autonomy is not limited to the patient but can extend to other family members (family autonomy).

At the level of clinical relationship with the patient, all interventions require informed, free, and expressed consent; consent is even considered imperative for professional ethics. Freedom in decision-making implies that the patient is truly autonomous to decide. Assuming that the patient is in full possession of their mental capacities (ethical competence), the freedom of will implies two points:

1   There is no coercion or external manipulation, especially no threat or suspected threat from any person, including healthcare professionals.
2   All conditions that may affect the patient's will are excluded, for example, the effects of medication, drugs, or alcohol, treatable affective disorders such as depression, or even intense pain and suffering.

In other words, the physician has the duty to inform the patient, in accessible language, all facts that are relevant for the patient to decide in full consciousness. Obviously, necessary prudence is required not only to inform but also to clarify issues with the patient in such a way that the transmitted information is comprehended with calmness and serenity. The greater the risk of the intervention, the greater the importance of obtaining valid and actual consent, although there are different possible modalities as follows (Nunes 2016):

1   Express consent: When informed consent is given actively (not tacitly) and orally within the context of a therapeutic alliance between the doctor and the patient.
2   Implied consent: When the intervention is implicit in the relationship between doctor and patient, and these individuals share a common goal.
3   Presumed consent: Consent is presumed when the minimum conditions for obtaining explicit consent are not met, and there is no objective and reliable information that the patient will object to a specific intervention, for example, emergency medical situations.
4   Written consent: In an environment of increasing judicial litigation and sustained increase in civil and criminal liability for damages, material evidence must be obtained proving that consent has been obtained.
5   Witnessed consent: This is an increase in the evidence that consent was effectively delivered. The witness may be a family member, friend, or healthcare professional other than the attending physician.
6   Generic consent: When the amount of information to be provided to the patient or their family is of enormous proportion, true informed consent is not feasible. It has been used in the context of performing genetic tests for numerous diseases and susceptibilities, such as multiplex genetic testing.
7   Family consent: In some cases, the patient is unable to provide explicit consent, for example, newborns, children, mentally ill patients, or patients in a persistent vegetative state. In these circumstances and within the limits of the best interests of the patient, the right of the family (or of the legitimate representative) to make medical decisions that are beneficial to the patient is usually recognized.
8   Therapeutic privilege: In exceptional circumstances, the physician can invoke therapeutic privilege to escape the responsibility of obtaining informed

consent. These circumstances refer to the existence of a high probability of physical or mental harm and not the mere emotional upset that can result from presenting the truth, for example, risk of heart attack or epileptic seizure.

In fact, a pluralistic society is based on citizens' ability to make free choices within a culture of responsibility and active citizenship (Nussbaum 1998). Note that the enshrinement of rights may imply the existence of correlative duties, deserving a comprehensive and detailed approach. This is perhaps one of the major gaps in many liberal democracies. Citizens are progressively aware of their rights, such as freedom of expression and association, but have not developed a parallel system of values that is reflected in the exercise of responsible citizenship. Therefore, it is not surprising that health system users only see themselves as rights holders in the same way that health professionals do not often perceive the duty to account for their activities (public accountability).

When there is a conflict between the parents' will and the best interests of the child, the *right to an open future* should be considered. This right indicates that children have the moral and legal right to the future exercise of autonomy, which falls within the general category of rights of the child (or another person with reduced capacity) that must be protected at present to be exercised later in life. This concept was proposed by Joel Feinberg in 1980 in the sense of rights-in-trust (Feinberg 1980). In the case of adolescents, the fundamental ethical question lies in the degree of assessed maturity. Therefore, consent or refusal of treatment must be strictly dependent on the assessment made in this regard (professional and legal assessment).

However, if any citizen has the right to be informed about a disease, they also have the right not to be informed about their health. This indicates that the exercise of autonomy may require contemplating exceptions to express consent if that is the real will of the patient (Newman 2015). Knowledge of personal genetic information or serology for human immunodeficiency virus (HIV) is a concrete example of this *right of not to know*. That is, there may be circumstances in which the physician must refrain from informing the patient if this is the patient's express wish (waivers) in accordance with the ethical principle of non-maleficence. Excessive and/or unwanted information can be clearly harmful to the patient. Therefore, physicians often provide such information to the family if this is the patient's wish. In this way, the right to personal self-determination is respected (Bode and Jones 2017).

However, freedom, autonomy, and self-determination are concepts that are clearly associated with privacy. This right is intended to restrict any external intrusion, presupposing, and noninterference in the intimate sphere of the person, among other circumstances. Privacy and confidentiality of health data imply the strict observance of professional secrecy by all agents involved in the processing of personal, biological, and/or genetic data, besides scrupulous archiving of the individual clinical records, regardless of the way in which data are stored (conventional or digital). Digitalization of clinical records is one of the most important measures of the modernization of the healthcare system but must be accompanied by necessary precautions so that patients' right to privacy is not violated. Considering that information systems can bring several benefits to patients, their families, and society at large, the implementation of an intranet may jeopardize the right to individual privacy. Therefore, measures should be taken to limit unauthorized access to private information. In specific circumstances, the *right to be forgotten* is a solution to preserve individual privacy and personal identity, leading to an erasure of personal data from digital networks (Correia et al. 2021).

One possible solution is to implement protection mechanisms for access to digital data, including the creation of complex keywords at different levels that limit access to the patient, their family (with consent), or to the healthcare staff directly involved in the patient's care. However, this situation is considerably aggravated by the generalization of big data-associated universal access (World Health Organization 2019). The idea of big data is one of the great challenges of global society that goes beyond healthcare because the protection of sensitive personal data is a right that is progressively valued by different communities. An example of this evolution is EU's General Data Protection Regulation (European Union 2016).

Respecting the previously expressed wishes of the patient is also a variant of the principle of autonomy, specifically, the wishes that are conveyed by family members, or those expressed in an advanced directive (Nunes 2017). A living will is a paradigmatic example of a previously expressed wish that has been already implemented in most modern countries (Burlá et al. 2014). More precisely, it corresponds to testamentary clauses on life since its effects refer to the period before death, contrary to what happens with conventional wills. By embracing the right to individual self-determination, the living will has been progressively considered in many countries as an instrument of manifestation of will. The main concern is the patient's right to withhold or withdraw extraordinary and futile treatments, such as assisted ventilation. The Convention for the Protection of Human Rights and Dignity of the Human Being with Regard to the Application of Biology and Medicine states in Article 9 that "The previously expressed wishes relating to a medical intervention by a patient who is not, at the time of the intervention, in a state to express his or her wishes shall be taken into account" (Council of Europe 1996). However, physicians are sometimes reluctant to respect a living will, especially in written form, because this will may question the best interests of the patient. However, there is no doubt that in many countries, this type of document is gaining acceptance in society and a specific law does exist to regulate its implementation.

In summary, there is a substantial paradigm shift in the provision of healthcare, particularly with the emergence of rights to individual self-determination and privacy. In addition, these rights have a double meaning: a) on the one hand, protection of intimacy, and b) on the other hand, the right of access to what is private and therefore, to the personal information that healthcare professionals must preserve by always respecting the exercise of personal freedom and the right to choose.

The Principle of Nondiscrimination

Basic rights also refer to the ethical imperative of equal treatment of all people before the law and social institutions. Thus, the principle of nondiscrimination becomes a fundamental driver of intersocial relations and is an essential factor in the construction of any liberal democracy. According to the UN's Committee on Economic, Social and Cultural Rights, the principle of nondiscrimination

> seeks to guarantee that human rights are exercised without discrimination of any kind based on race, color, sex, language, religion, political or other opinion, national or social origin, property, birth, or other status such as disability, age, marital and family status, sexual orientation, and gender identity, health status, place of residence, economic and social situation.
>
> (Committee on Economic, Social and Cultural Rights 2009)

In fact, within this framework of secular pluralism, another important right of the patient is not being discriminated against or stigmatized by arbitrary characteristics. The right to nondiscrimination and non-stigmatization is an important achievement of modern civilization, making any discriminatory practice ethically reprehensible since it violates the right to a person's self-determination (Engelhardt 1996). In healthcare, nondiscrimination is important in different settings. Some instances are described below.

1 Genetic data: There is a possibility of discriminatory practices in genetics, which should be avoided. For example, the emergence of genetic technology has the potential to subtly stigmatize a particular class of people. Through stigmatization, if the aim is to mark, label, or discredit someone or a community because of a special characteristic, the generalization of genetic testing may then reflect and even reinforce society's negative attitudes toward individual's with a disability or a simple genetic change (Melo and Nunes 2000). Moreover, genetic technology allows some deficiencies to be socially considered as a matter of choice rather than destiny. This tendency should be avoided by reinforcing the notion that quality of life is independent of any genetic determinism and that the life of a person with a disability is worthwhile. Society should allocate the resources necessary for effective equal opportunity for people with disabilities (health, education, and employment). Citizens' rights, namely the rights of handicapped people, are the true spirit of a liberal democracy, that is, the primacy of the person. This perspective is in accordance with the principle of reproductive autonomy and the legal rights of couples to make procreative choices. This means that in a fair society, a balance should be reached between rights and duties and that the rights to life and self-determination of handicapped people should also be considered.

2 Gender discrimination: Gender equality can be understood as the creation of conditions for men and women to have the same situations to enjoy their rights and to contribute to and benefit from social, economic, cultural, and

political developments. It indicates society's equal appreciation of the similarities and differences between men and women and their respective social roles. In other words, it is intended that men and women are balanced partners in the family and community in general. Moreover, this perspective is subscribed to by most international conventions in this field and recognizes the importance of diversity between the sexes. This is because each person must be free to assure self-fulfillment and to make the choices that they deem most appropriate. Gender equality has come a long way in all societies, but significant barriers must still be overcome regarding access to health, especially reproductive health, education, and health education. However, there is an important generational evolution in this matter. Younger generations are looking for an equitable distribution of family functions and tasks because women have progressively assumed their place in the labor market and in society in general, namely in politics and business. Therefore, it is natural for younger families to reconcile work, family, and personal life. Innovative measures are also needed in this situation that are adjusted to each social and cultural reality to ensure that in terms of access to healthcare, all existing gaps relating to the gender of patients are corrected (Nunes 2020).

3   Human research: Discriminatory practices may also exist in human research. The priority of the individual's interests, especially when the person is vulnerable and ill, over the interests of science and society recalls the primacy of the human being and their dignity as the foundation of a pluralistic society. Moreover, this concept helps materialize the intrinsic and noninstrumental values of the human individual. The primacy of human beings over science is of relevance in scientific research, particularly in clinical trials of pharmaceuticals for human use. This provision is established in existing national and international laws and guidelines on this subject so that clinical trials can only be carried out on human beings when the results of laboratory testing show that the risks to the person to be tested on are proportional to the benefits (ethical principle of non-maleficence). One of the main responsibilities of ethics committees is to weigh the risks and benefits considering the best interests of the subject. As an instrument of a modern society which seeks to defend the legitimate rights of patients without reservations, ethics committees are an important tool for intra-institutional regulation and anti-discriminatory practices, particularly regarding research on human subjects (National Commission for the Protection of Human Subjects of Biomedical and Behavioral Research 1978). Although society has a social interest in the advancement of scientific knowledge and in the technological evolution of biomedicine, it should also promote equal access to all potential beneficiaries of clinical research results (Nunes 2003). As scientific research is carried out on a global scale, so the benefits must also be universal (Boman and Kruse 2017).

4   Spiritual care: In a pluralistic and tolerant society, the right to spiritual support and religious assistance, as a patient's option, seems fundamental. Although there is a clear separation between the state and the church in

liberal democracies, the right to personal self-determination is the backbone of democracy. Therefore, patients' spiritual support is of special relevance in the hospital context. This assistance reflects the fact that the human being, enjoying personal freedom, is a relational being living collectively (Rego and Nunes 2019). Unconditional respect for this right can be achieved by guaranteeing freedom of conscience and religion to all patients in the healthcare system by offering the possibility of spiritual and religious identification, regulating this assistance in all healthcare services, promoting the existence of physical spaces (places of worship) and financial resources for this purpose, and sensitizing healthcare professionals to the existence of this right. It is a new vision of social responsibility to ensure the full exercise of this right (Brandão et al. 2013).

As noted, there are different ways in which patients can be subject to discrimination in the healthcare system, whether by disease or disability, system inefficiencies, gender or social condition, or the way science is organized on a global scale. Besides the existence of adequate legislation and the creation of effective IRAs that control these practices, one way of preventing discrimination in the healthcare system is to give all patients the opportunity to show their discomfort about the way healthcare was delivered.

The evolution of healthcare systems worldwide has been accompanied by citizens' awareness of their rights and duties, particularly regarding the existence of effective accountability mechanisms, and complaints and claims (Nunes et al. 2009). A complaint should be viewed as an instrument of performance improvement in any healthcare organization. Indeed, there is an increase in complaints and legal proceedings for moral damage and personality rights. That is, it is often not a matter of professional malpractice or medical negligence but only of deficient human relationships. This complaint system implies a substantial change in the healthcare system from the perspective of its humanization.

Personality rights are increasingly valued in this context. Medical and other healthcare professionals should acquire specific empathic skills. Indeed, a good professional practice should value not only technical competence but also *soft skills* that enable professionals to deal with human suffering.

Conclusion

Since the proclamation of the Universal Declaration of Human Rights by the UN General Assembly in Paris on December 10, 1948 (United Nations 1948), the international movement around the progressive recognition of basic rights inherent to the human condition has been developing in all societies, albeit at varying rates. In addition, the development of robust democracies with effective social and political institutions is a decisive factor for a new world order based on peace, multilateral cooperation, and sustainable development.

Democracy and human rights have also enabled us to view health as a collective goal of humanity and to implement transnational global health initiatives to improve health levels without looking at historically determined geographical boundaries (Bulc et al. 2019). A global health vision implies the progressive consideration of a universal right to healthcare, indicating the right to access healthcare of appropriate quality.

However, the existence and implementation of a universal right to healthcare implies that other rights are also respected, namely, the right to self-determination, the right to privacy, and the universal principle of nondiscrimination. Specific measures should be implemented to accomplish this goal. These rights are especially valued in many contemporary societies since the feeling of relative justice contributes decisively to personal self-realization. Therefore, every effort must be made by different social actors, including governments, professional associations, nongovernmental organizations, and private companies, to create a planetary awareness of the importance of human rights in general and specifically of the universal right to healthcare.

References

Arendt H. 1995. *Qu'est-ce que la politique? Texte établi par Ursula Ludz*. Essais, Éditions du Seuil, Paris.

Beauchamp T and Childress J. 2013. *Principles of biomedical ethics*. Oxford University Press, New York, 7th edition.

Beddow A. 2017. Immanuel Kant and the myth of perpetual peace. *The National Interest*, August 28. https://nationalinterest.org/feature/immanuel-kant-the-myth-perpetual-peace-22087.

Bessette J. 1981. Deliberative democracy: The majority principle in republican government. *How democratic is the constitution?* R Goldwin and W Shambra (Editors). American Enterprise Institute, Washington, DC.

Bode L and Jones ML. 2017. Ready to forget: American attitudes toward the right to be forgotten. *Information Society* 33 (2): 76–85. DOI: 10.1080/01972243.2016.1271071.

Bollyky T, Templin T, Cohen M, Schoder D, Dieleman J and Wigley S. 2019. The relationships between democratic experience, adult health, and cause-specific mortality in 170 countries between 1980 and 2016: An observational analysis. *The Lancet* 393 (10181): 1628–1640. DOI: 10.1016/S0140-6736(19)30235-1.

Boman M and Kruse E. 2017. Supporting global health goals with information and communications technology. *Global Health Action* 10 (3): 6–13.

Brandão C, Rego G, Duarte I and Nunes R. 2013. Social responsibility: A new paradigm of hospital governance? *Health Care Analysis* 21 (4): 390–402.

Buchanan D. 2000. *An ethic for health promotion. Rethinking the sources of human wellbeing*. Oxford University Press, New York.

Bulc B, Al-Wahdani B, Bustreo F et al. 2019. Urgency for transformation: Youth engagement in global health. *The Lancet* 7: 1–2.

Burlá C, Rego G and Nunes R. 2014. Alzheimer, dementia and the living will: A proposal. *Medicine, Health Care and Philosophy* 17 (3): 389–395.

Capon A and Corvalana C. 2018. Climate change and health: Global issue, local responses. *Public Health Research & Practice* 28 (4): 1–3.

Caranti L. 2016. Kantian peace and liberal peace: Three concerns. *The Journal of Political Philosophy* 24 (4): 446–469. https://onlinelibrary.wiley.com/doi/abs/10.1111/jopp.12097.

CIOMS – Council for International Organizations of Medical Sciences. 1997. *Ethics, equity and health for all*, Z. Bankowski, J. Bryant and J. Gallagher (Editors). CIOMS, Geneva.

Committee on Economic, Social and Cultural Rights. 2009. *General comment N° 20, Non-discrimination in economic, social and cultural rights.* Economic and Social Council, United Nations, Geneva.

Correia M, Rego G and Nunes R. 2021. Gender transition: Is there a right to be forgotten. *Health Care Analysis* 2021 (29): 283–300.

Council of Europe. 1996. *Convention for the protection of human rights and dignity of the human being with regard to the application of biology and medicine.* Council of Europe, Strasbourg, November.

Dworkin R. 2000. *Sovereign virtue. The theory and practice of equality.* Harvard University Press, Cambridge, MA.

Engelhardt HT. 1996. *The foundations of bioethics.* Oxford University Press, New York, 2nd edition.

European Union. 2016. General data protection regulation. Regulation (EU) 2016/679 of the European parliament and of the council of 27 April 2016 on the protection of natural persons with regard to the processing of personal data and on the free movement of such data. http://eur-lex.europa.eu/legal-content/PT/TXT/?uri=CELEX:32016R0679.

Feinberg J. 1980. The child's right to an "open future" in whose child? *Children's rights, parental authority and state power*, W Aiken and H LaFollette (Editors). Littlefield, Adams & Co, Totowa, NJ.

Habermas J. 1997. *Droit et démocracie. Entre faits et normes.* NRF Essais, Galimard, Paris.

Institute for Health Metrics and Evaluation. 2019. Global study highlights role of democracy in improving adult health. www.healthdata.org/news-release/global-study-highlights-role-democracy-improving-adult-health.

Jia P and Wang Y. 2019. Global health efforts and opportunities related to the belt and road initiative. *The Lancet* 7: 703–705.

Majone G. 1997. From the positive to the regulatory state. *Journal of Public Policy* 17 (2): 139–167.

McLuhan M and Powers B. 1989. *Chapter 1: The resonating interval in the global village. transformations in world life and media in the 21st century.* Oxford University Press, Oxford.

Melo H and Nunes R 2000. Genetic testing in the workplace: Medical, ethical and legal issues. *Law and the Human Genome Review* 13: 119–142.

National Commission for the Protection of Human Subjects of Biomedical and Behavioral Research. 1978. *The Belmont report. Ethical principles and guidelines for the protection of human subjects of research.* Government Printing Office (DHEW publication No. (OS) 78–0012), Washington, DC.

Newman AL. 2015. What the "right to be forgotten" means for privacy in a digital age. *Science* 347 (6221): 507–508.

Nunes R. 2003. Evidence-based medicine: A new tool for resource allocation? *Medicine, Health Care and Philosophy* 6 (3): 297–301.

Nunes R. 2016. *Diretivas antecipadas de vontade.* Conselho Federal de Medicina, Brasília.

Nunes R. 2017. *Ensaios em bioética.* Conselho Federal de Medicina, Brasília.

Nunes R. 2020. Addressing gender inequality to promote basic human rights and development: A global perspective. *CEDIS Working Papers* 2020 (1). http://cedis.fd.unl.pt/blog/project/addressing-gender-inequality-to-promote-basic-human-rights-and-development-a-global-perspective/.

Nunes R, Brandão C and Rego G. 2011. Public accountability and sunshine healthcare regulation. *Health Care Analysis* 19 (4): 352–364.

Nunes R, Nunes SB and Rego G. 2017. Healthcare as a universal right. *Journal of Public Health* 25: 1–9.

Nunes R and Rego G. 2014. Priority setting in health care: A complementary approach. *Health Care Analysis* 22: 292–303.

Nunes R, Rego G and Brandão C. 2009. Healthcare regulation as a tool for public accountability. *Medicine, Health Care and Philosophy* 12: 257–264.

Nussbaum MC. 1998. The good as discipline, the good as freedom. *The ethics of consumption and global stewardship*, D Crocker (Editor). Rowman and Littlefield, Lanham, MA.

Rego MF and Nunes R. 2019. The interface between psychology and spirituality in palliative care. *Journal of Health Psychology* 24 (3): 279–287.

Sen A. 1999. *Development as freedom*. Knopf, New York.

Simão M, Wirtz V, Al-Ansary L et al. 2018. A global accountability mechanism for access to essential medicines. *The Lancet* 392: 2418–2420.

UNESCO. 2005. Universal declaration of bioethics and human rights. www.unesco.org/new/en/social-and-human-sciences/themes/bioethics/bioethics-and-human-rights/.

United Nations. 1948. Universal declaration of human rights. Proclaimed by the United Nations General Assembly in Paris on 10 December 1948, General Assembly resolution 217 A.

Watts N, Amann M, Arnell N et al. 2018. The 2018 report of the lancet countdown on health and climate change: Shaping the health of nations for centuries to come. *The Lancet* 392: 2479–2514.

World Health Organization. 2019. *WHO guideline recommendations on digital interventions for health system strengthening*. World Health Organization, Geneva. License: CC BY-NC-SA 3.0 IGO.

Index

Note: Page numbers in *italic* indicate a figure and page numbers in **bold** indicate a box on the corresponding page.

For Product Safety Concerns and Information please contact our EU
representative GPSR@taylorandfrancis.com
Taylor & Francis Verlag GmbH, Kaufingerstraße 24, 80331 München, Germany

www.ingramcontent.com/pod-product-compliance
Lightning Source LLC
Chambersburg PA
CBHW060304220326
41598CB00027B/4226

9 781032 193250